The Medical Consultation:
A practical guide for hospital specialists

BJHM Occasional Series

Other books in the series

Contemporary Psychiatry by Dr K Katz

BJHM Occasional Series

The Medical Consultation:

A practical guide for hospital specialists

by
David Short

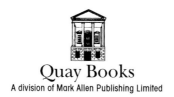

Quay Books
A division of Mark Allen Publishing Limited

Quay Books Division of Mark Allen Publishing Limited
Jesses Farm, Snow Hill, Dinton, Nr Salisbury, Wilts, SP3 5HN

©Mark Allen Publishing Ltd, 1995

British Library Cataloguing-in-Publication Data
A catalogue record for this book is available from the British Library

ISBN 1-85642-118-X

Printed in the UK by Biddles Limited, Woodbridge Park Estate,
Guildford, Surrey, GU1 1DA

CONTENTS

ACKNOWLEDGEMENTS

In writing this book, I recognise a debt to three categories of people: teachers, facilitators and practical advisers.

Among my teachers, I think particularly of Dr Evan Bedford, physician to the Middlesex Hospital, Dr William Evans, cardiologist to the London Hospital and Dr Wallace Brigden, physician to the London Hospital.

My great facilitator has been my wife to whom I owe and incalculable debt for providing me with a happy and relatively stress-free home life, and for undertaking the main burden of caring for our family.

My advisers are primarily my colleagues in Aberdeen, who kindly read and commented on some of the chapters of the book, although without assuming responsibility for what I have written. Dr Alan Johnston reviewed chapter 8, Dr Peter Brunt, chapter 11 and Dr Leslie Stankler, chapters 13 and 15.

I have also received helpful practical advice and encouragement from Professor Alan Johnson of Sheffield, Dr Paul Buxton of Edinburgh and Dr Andrew Fergusson of London. I am indebted to my friend John Lonsdale for checking the proofs.

Finally, I must acknowledge the great helpfulness and skill of Ms Valery Moran, Publisher at Quay Books Division of Mark Allen Publishing Group, in preparing this book for publication.

FOREWORD

This is a book which, I believe, fills a major gap. A recent conference on `Medicine's core values' — described as the first `summit' meeting of the profession since 1961 — emphasised the centrality of the consultation. Much has been written about general practice consultation but virtually nothing about specialist consultation, which is in many ways quite different.

This book is timely because things are changing. The patient is no longer willing to accept a paternalistic, doctor-knows-best attitude. He (or she) wants to ask questions and discuss the proposed treatment. Nor are patients satisfied with a medical approach which focuses almost entirely on physical abnormalities. If the drift to alternative medicine tells us anything, it is that the patient is looking for a consultation in which he is treated as a person and not as a disease. How this may be approached in practice is indicated in the chapter on `Total patient care'. Although the advances in medical and surgical technology inspire admiration for medical scientists, they may easily induce fear rather than trust.

Another reason why this book is timely is because medical consultation is in the process of being transformed by rapid developments in information technology. The advances in diagnosis and prognosis resulting from computer assistance is the background to the chapter on `The science and art of diagnosis'. Also, the consultant is less and less a solo performer. His relationship with his assistants and back-room staff is the subject of the chapter on `Team care'.

David Short is exceptionally well qualified to write on this subject in view of the breadth of his experience. He spent ten years as a junior doctor in Bristol and London, and had the opportunity of working with some of the greatest diagnostic and investigative physicians in the Middlesex, Royal London and National Heart hospitals. In Aberdeen, he developed the unusual custom of going on the rounds of some of his colleagues, to observe and learn from their practice.

Soon after his appointment as a general physician with cardiological interest in Aberdeen, he inaugurated the post-graduate teaching programme. Later, he pioneered a programme of medical audit for the division of medicine. Although private practice constituted only a small fraction of his work, it did mean that he was familiar with the whole gamut of clinical experience.

Before his retirement, Dr Short was given a personal chair, specifically designated as a professorship in *clinical* medicine. He was already chairman of the ethics committee of the University of Aberdeen and the Grampian Health Board and Physician to the Queen in Scotland.

This book is important not only for consultants in all specialties, but also for those on the promotion ladder, and especially for those involved in training the doctors of the future. Developments in the organisation of medical care involve doctors in spending a greater proportion of their time on committees, organising their business plans and contracts, and less with their patients. But it is certain that, whatever changes may come, the consultation with an individual patient will remain at the heart of any system of medical care.

by Lord McColl, MS FRCS FACS

PREFACE

The supreme importance of the consultation

The consultation is the foundation of medical practice. The conference held at the end of 1994 in the British Medical Association House, London, to consider Core Values for the medical profession in the 21st Century gave as its first conclusion:

The personal consultation should remain the bedrock of medical practice.

Although the practice of medicine is changing continuously with advances in knowledge, technical developments in diagnosis and treatment, and the relentless increase in regulation, the essence of medical practice remains the same; namely, the consultation between a patient in need and a doctor with the power to help. This heart of the transaction has never been better expressed than by Sir James Spence:

> `The essential unit of medical practice is the occasion when, in the intimacy of the consulting room or sick room, a person who is ill or believes himself to be ill, seeks the advice of a doctor whom he trusts.`[1]

(Spence was fortunate in living in an age in which the masculine pronoun was generally accepted as embracing the female of the species on an equal footing. I adopt the same convention, as a matter of convenience.)

The theme of the medical consultation is therefore lastingly relevant and important. Whatever developments may take place in the pattern of medical care in the future — for example, whether the consultant moves into the community instead of being based in hospital — makes no fundamental difference to the essence of the consultation

It may be asked, 'Has not more than enough already been written on this subject?' The answer is that although a great deal has been written about consultation in general practice, remarkably little has been written about specialist consultation. The two are very different. I am writing here against the background of the British system in which every patient has a general practitioner or primary care physician, who has a broad knowledge of disease. He deals with most of the patient's needs himself, and refers others to specialists under the National Health Service or privately, as appropriate.

The difference between specialist and GP consultation

One major difference between general practice and specialist consultation is that the general practitioner is commonly dealing with what may be called an 'undifferentiated' problem. Many studies have indicated that upwards of a quarter of his patients present with problems of major or minor psycho-pathology. The specialist, on the other hand, has the advantage of dealing with a more defined problem. Many patients come to the consultant specifically for the elucidation of signs which the general practitioner has noticed, such as a lump or a cardiac murmur, or a symptom such as headache or dyspnoea. Another important difference is that the general practitioner usually has the advantage of a more intimate knowledge of his patient's background and environment. The specialist knows the disease; the general practitioner knows the patient.

Having emphasised the fundamental difference between specialist and general practice, it must be admitted that some of the recent insights pointing the way to better general practice are undoubtedly relevant to specialist consultation. This applies particularly to the recognition of the pervasive role of the mind in a great deal of illness, and the importance of exploring this dimension by asking open-ended questions. Specialists also need to

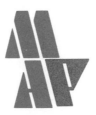

MARK ALLEN PUBLISHING LIMITED

Circulation & Subscriptions Department,
Jesses Farm, Snow Hill, Dinton,
Salisbury, Wiltshire SP3 5HN

Telephone 01722 716997 Facsimile 01722 716926

with compliments

be alert to the danger of regarding the discovery of a minor physical abnormality as being necessarily the basis of the patient's symptoms. This may seem a superfluous warning, but it is a fact that many patients with mild symptoms without any physical basis have had their attention focused on their heart because of an unimportant murmur or the presence of extrasystoles, or on their colon because of an irrelevant finding on examination or investigation. There is, in fact, nothing really new in these insights. They were well understood by former generations of doctors, but they have become submerged by the rising tide of medical science, with its emphasis on physical abnormalities and the desire of many patients to know every detail about their condition.

An orthopaedic specialist, newly elevated to consultant status, exclaimed: 'The orthopaedics is no problem, but no one taught me how to be a consultant.' This book is designed to go some way towards filling that need; focusing on the specialist consultation itself. I am not concerned about specific specialist interests; how to be an expert cardiologist or neurologist or gynaecologist. There is plenty written about these subjects. What I am concerned about here, is factors common to all specialties: how to be a good consultant.

Medical consultation can be a bore or a delight: a chore or an occasion of pleasure and profit. My hope is that this book will help new consultants and those in training to approach outpatient clinics with a sense of anticipation and also help them to avoid some of the pitfalls which lie in wait for the unprepared.

This book makes no attempt to cover legal aspects of medical practice or to offer advice on consultants' contracts or on disciplinary complaints and sickness procedures, all of which are well-covered by BMA publications.

Reference

1.   Spence J (1960) *The purpose and practice of medicine.* OUP, London: 273-4

Chapter 1
WHAT THE PATIENT IS LOOKING FOR

- ◆ Reasons for general practitioner referral to a specialist
- ◆ Communication
- ◆ Confidentiality

It is important that the consultant should not only make a correct diagnosis and give sound advice, but also satisfy the patient. It is necessary, therefore, to understand the patient's expectations.

Patients attend specialists for various reasons. Most come because they have noticed disquieting symptoms or apparent abnormalities. Some come at the insistence of their spouse. Others come because a recent death has reminded them that they have a bad family history. In British practice, most patients who attend specialists have been referred by a general practitioner.

General practitioners refer patients to specialists basically for one of three reasons. The commonest is some degree of uncertainty regarding diagnosis or treatment. The next commonest, and this sometimes overlaps the first, is to satisfy the patient. The third reason for referral is to silence someone who is causing trouble. In a city with a large medical centre, the general practitioner will select the specialist he thinks best suited to the patient. It will not always be the one with the greatest diagnostic flair. It is often the one he thinks will reassure the patient. It was said that doctors referred patients to Lord Dawson of Penn, the physician to the royal family, primarily because he made them feel better.

It is true to say that almost every patient considers his complaint to be one of great peculiarity or perhaps obscurity, demanding prompt attention[1]. He views the first consultation with a medical specialist as a momentous event. Health is so important, and disease so mysterious and ominous to the layman, that patients cannot be blamed for being apprehensive.

Two main criteria

What are patients hoping for? They have two main criteria by which they judge a consultation. Ultimately, they look for a diagnosis and some idea of the prognosis. The two most important questions from the patient's point of view are 'What is the name of the illness from which I am suffering?' and 'Is it serious?' A diagnosis of 'Nothing wrong' may be medically correct but, by itself, is no answer to the patient's prime question. Even if the patient has come purely for reassurance, he still wants an explanation. He wants to know what caused the symptom for which he went to the doctor in the first place. If the chest pain did not arise in the heart, what was its cause?

The second criterion by which a patient judges a consultation is good communication. Did the doctor listen well? Did he volunteer information and explanation? Did he give me time to ask questions? Patients express more dissatisfaction with the information they receive (or fail to receive) than with any other aspect of medical care. There is abundant evidence for this statement, and it makes sobering reading.

In a survey of 400 patients recently discharged from hospital, 65% saw communication with medical personnel as the least satisfactory aspect of their hospital stay. Among 292 patients who had made their first visit to a specialist in the preceding six months, nearly a quarter said that they were not given any information unless they asked for it. Two-thirds said that they felt the specialist seemed too busy, and that there was not enough time for questions[2]. Lack of communication is given as one of the main reasons for patients going to alternative practitioners. The patient feels the need to be listened to, to be treated with respect, and to be given full, unhurried, jargon-free explanations.

The consensus of many surveys is that the patient is looking first and foremost for a doctor who is conscientious, caring, unselfish and a good listener. He wants to feel that he is safe in the doctor's hands and that the doctor will be pleasant, considerate and, above all, competent. He will not be satisfied or impressed for long merely by 'a good bedside manner'.

Other expectations

The patient is also looking for absolute confidentiality. He expects that what he tells the doctor will not be passed on to anyone else without his permission. Balint[3] told the story of a registrar who was taking a woman's history, and trying to discover the cause of her depression. The patient was unforthcoming. Finally, she broke down crying: *"I can't tell you. I won't tell you. I told it to my doctor in the last hospital, and the next day the whole hospital knew it."*

It is essential, if an accurate diagnosis is to be made, that patients disclose to us all the facts which may be relevant to the diagnosis. Since, by definition, patients cannot know which facts are relevant or irrelevant, the doctor must gently persuade them to reveal as much about themselves as possible. The more information the doctor has, the more reliable the diagnosis is likely to be. But unless doctors can be trusted to keep it confidential, patients will not reveal it and the quality of their care will suffer[4].

It must be added that not all patients go to see a specialist with such a straightforward medical objective. Some go because they are lonely and want companionship. They want someone to talk to, and they hope to find this need met in the doctor or the receptionist or the other patients in the waiting room. This is particularly true, in my experience, of a considerable proportion of patients being followed up in hospital outpatient clinics.

Some go to the doctor to look for sympathy. To hear someone important say *"I think you are wonderful, the way you carry on"* is music to their ears. Others go to the doctor to get medical backing for their own views. They find their work a strain, and it is a triumph to be able to say to the boss: *"The doctor says my work is too heavy for me."* A few rich patients go to see specialists so as to be able to boast about it: *"Of course, I am one of Professor Snook's special patients."* Such motives are often cleverly concealed and it may be some time into the consultation before the doctor realises that he is wasting his time.

References

1. Longcope WT (1962) Methods and medicine. In: Davenport WH, ed. *The Good Physician*. Macmillan Co, New York: 558

2. Pendleton D (1983) Doctor–patient communications: A review. In: Pendleton D, Hasler J, eds. *Doctor-Patient Communication*. Academic Press, London: 30

3. Balint M (1961) The pyramid and the psychotherapeutic relationship. *Lancet* **ii**: 1051–4

4. Horner JS (1994) Confidentiality. *Nucleus* **April**: 2–8

Chapter 2
FIRST IMPRESSIONS — BOTH WAYS

◆ The impression conveyed by the patient to the doctor
◆ The impression conveyed by the doctor to the patient
◆ The use of a questionnaire
◆ Punctuality
◆ Dress
◆ How the doctor greets the patient

Dr William Evans, my old 'chief' at The Royal London Hospital, used to say:

"During a consultation there are two people at work. Whilst the doctor is searching for a diagnosis, the patient is quietly summing up the doctor. And it is often the patient who reaches his conclusion first!"

First impressions are important both to the doctor and to the patient. The doctor, particularly the physician, is trying to pick up initial clues to the nature of the patient's problem by observing facial appearance, colour, tone of voice, type of cough, tremor, odour, etc. He is also trying to assess the patient's attitude to his illness. The patient, for his part, is trying to decide whether the doctor is really interested in his problem.

First impressions are formed even before the doctor and patient meet. Most patients have heard something of the reputation of the doctor they have come to see, and perhaps about his life-style. Not so long ago, doctors used to try to impress patients by driving an expensive car or one with a personalised numberplate. I sense that patients are less impressed by these trappings now. That is certainly true of the inhabitants of northeast Scotland, where I live.

The patient's attitude towards the doctor is influenced not only by his reputation, but also by the reputation of the hospital or clinic and, indeed, of the medical profession in general. At the present time, the medical profession still carries considerable respect. This makes the doctor's task easier because he can assume a large measure of trust in the patient. In a survey of patients attending a general practitioner for the first time[1], it was found that many knew nothing of the doctor they were going to consult, and seemed unperturbed by this. Clearly they were prepared to rely on the reputation of the profession. This is, no doubt, equally true of patients seeing a specialist for the first time.

The attitude of the reception staff and the state of the waitingroom also convey impressions regarding the doctor. Patients notice the degree of respect shown by the receptionist, and the state of the waiting room and its furnishings. In private practice, the consultant can include personal touches, such as lining the shelves of the waiting room with impressive books and perhaps displaying certificates of diplomas they have been awarded. Such individualism is impossible in a hospital clinic, where the consultation suite is used by many doctors.

Questionnaires

Some doctors make use of questionnaires, to be filled in by the patient before the consultation. I did this myself latterly. The preamble made it clear that the purpose of the questionnaire was not primarily to save the doctor's time, but an attempt to cover the inevitable forgetfulness that patients experience when trying to answer questions 'off the cuff'.

The preface carried the explanation: 'It is often difficult when you see a doctor to remember all the things you were meaning to tell him.' It then provided a series of headings offering a framework for the patient to give the history of the present and previous illnesses with dates, an opportunity to list any drugs he was taking, and space to mention other problems, such as depression, worries, etc[2]. Some consider questionnaires to be a bad introduction to a consultation, but in my experience none of the patients objected and a few positively welcomed it as an indication of the thoroughness of the specialist's approach. I certainly found questionnaires helpful.

Punctuality

Busy patients dislike being kept waiting, although most realise that doctors may be delayed by emergencies of various kinds and cannot regulate their lives precisely. Patients certainly deserve an explanation of any appreciable delay. Although punctuality is important, it is not all-important. Most patients would greatly prefer a satisfying consultation, involving a considerable delay, to one which is punctual but perfunctory. It must be added that some patients, particularly those who are lonely, are quite unconcerned about delays. They enjoy passing the time chatting to other patients, to the receptionist or to the nurse.

Dress

Dress is important — and controversial. We live in an age, at least in Britain, when informality is in vogue, and smartness and tidiness are disparaged. But dress conveys a message to the patient. Dr Solomon Papper[3] tells the story of an unkempt drug addict whom he admitted to his ward. The patient saw one of the students who looked untidy and scruffy, and angrily refused to allow him to touch him or participate in his care, calling him a 'slob'.

The whole issue of dress centres on its effect on the patient, particularly with regard to the confidence he places in his doctor. Most patients expect a doctor to look like a traditional doctor and follow the standard set by nurses, who are almost always correctly and neatly turned out.

In a recent survey of Scottish patients' attitudes to doctors' dress[4], patients were asked to look at photographs of doctors dressed in clothing of various degrees of formality and mark them in order of preference. A smart dark suit was acceptable, as was a tweed jacket, but an open collar, short sleeves or jeans were not acceptable. A female doctor was most appreciated if she wore a white coat over a sweater, blouse and skirt. The wearing of a white coat was not universally respected. Patients in higher social classes appreciated it, especially on women doctors, but those in lower income groups seemed wary of it. Although this was a survey of attitudes to general practitioners, it may also reflect attitudes to hospital doctors.

Another argument in favour of the white coat is that it is a symbol of cleanliness and professionalism. When wearing a white coat, the doctor is permitted to carry out examinations that would otherwise have been rejected. On the other hand, many paediatricians believe that not wearing a white coat makes them less frightening to children. Fashions change, but the principle of helping and not hindering the doctor–patient relationship remains paramount.

Greeting the patient

The patient should be welcomed with a smile and, if appropriate, a handshake. If the doctor is distracted by a telephone call, or is jotting down notes on another matter, he should apologise to the patient and promise to give him his full attention as soon as he is ready. Patients have told me that they found it reassuring to be addressed by name, for example *"Good morning, Mrs A"*, rather than *"Now, who are you?"* or (aside to the receptionist or assistant) *"Who is this patient?"*

Should patients be addressed by surname or by first name? The current trend is to call patients by their first name. Recent studies, in both London and Scotland, have shown that a majority of patients are happy with this practice, although a significant minority strongly object, particularly older patients and those from the higher social classes. The principle is that patients should be addressed in a way which demonstrates respect, equality and friendliness. My own practice was to be friendly but formal on first acquaintance, often changing to greater familiarity later. If in doubt, the patient should be asked: *"How do you like to be addressed?"*

It is important that doctors identify themselves. For this purpose, the practice of wearing a badge with the doctor's name in bold print, and the designation, e.g. consultant, registrar, etc, is to be strongly recommended.

All patients, especially women, like to be seen in an attractive light. Some doctors, in order to cut delay to a minimum, insist that their patients should be undressed and ready for examination before they see them. I believe this is bad psychology. The patient feels a loss of dignity, and this gets the doctor–patient relationship off to a bad start.

References

1. Salisbury C (1989) How do people choose their doctor? *Br Med J* **299**: 608–10

2. Short D (1986) Why don't we use questionnaires in the medical out-patient clinic? *Health Bull* **44**: 228–33

3. Papper S (1983) *Doing Right: Everyday Medical Ethics*. Little, Brown and Co, Boston: 125

4. McKinstry B, Wang J (1991) Putting on the style: what patients think of the way their doctor dresses. *Br J Gen Pract* **41**: 275–8

Chapter 3
HISTORY TAKING

◆ The supreme importance of the history
◆ Recognising diagnostic clues
◆ Creating a helpful atmosphere
◆ Really listening
◆ The doctor as detective
◆ Regional differences in symptomatology
◆ The doctor's questions

Unless the patient is unconscious, or *in extremis*, the first step in a consultation is naturally an invitation to the patient to explain why he has sought medical help, and to describe the symptom or symptoms which are causing concern.

The supreme importance of the history

The history can justifiably be regarded as the most important part of the consultation[1]. It has been shown to point to the correct diagnosis in one-half to well over three-quarters of cases, depending on the type of clinic.

Since much of the essential diagnostic information arises from the interview, it is obvious that history taking cannot safely be delegated. Moreover, the physician's ability to understand the patient's needs largely determines the patient's satisfaction with the consultation. This in turn increases compliance, and thus improves the health outcome. Rapport with the patient also reduces the risk of litigation, since the majority of malpractice allegations arise from a failure in communication.

To become effective listeners and communicators, doctors must master a defined body of knowledge, skills and attitudes. Clinical communication skills do not necessarily improve from mere experience[2]. They need to be repeatedly updated. Hence the importance of continuing medical education. The main areas that need to be learned are the structure and function of medical interviewing, and the elements of psychiatry in relation to medicine. Many specialists are weak in the recognition of diagnostic clues to depression, anxiety and 'somatisation' — the tendency to complain of physical symptoms which cannot be accounted for by pathological findings[3]. History taking is a sphere in which video recording and playback has been shown to improve performance.

Basic requirements

As a rule, the consultation should be completely private. Spence[4], in his lecture on 'The function of the hospital outpatient department', insisted that no nurses, social workers or other assistants should be allowed in the room. He permitted a maximum of two students to assist the consultant, with the patient's consent, and laid down that there should be no clinical teaching except between cases. Anyone who needed to enter the consulting room had to knock on the door.

It is important to give the patient one's full attention. Brigadier Hardy-Roberts[5], writing from the perspective of a secretary-superintendent of a London teaching hospital, gave valuable advice on what he called 'office manners'. Although his words were primarily directed at trainees in hospital administration, they are equally applicable to the doctor's relationship with his patient.

> `Avoid any appearance of hurrying him. Give him your entire attention, and let nothing seem to distract you. The telephone should be switched through to your secretary so that she can take the calls. ... If there is an urgent message for you, she should write it down and bring it in unobtrusively, so that you can glance at it when it is your turn to speak.'

This is in sharp contrast to the situation in many clinics, where doctors wander in and out of the consulting room, and telephone interruptions are accepted.

The position in which the doctor sits in relation to the patient is important. It has been shown that if the doctor and patient sit close to each other across the corner of the desk, there is six times more interaction than if they speak to each other across the desk[6].

Most patients who have been referred to a specialist assume that their general practitioner has given the consultant all the essential points in the history. They are understandably puzzled and not infrequently annoyed to have to go through it all again. It is therefore important for the consultant to explain the necessity for re-checking essential facts. If some weeks have elapsed between the writing of the general practitioner's letter and the consultation, he can explain that it is important to find out whether the situation has changed.

The aim of the doctor is to elicit the patient's complaints and then to elucidate them in terms of disordered bodily or mental function. Although this sounds simple, diagnosis is a difficult art, especially in the case of rare diseases and diseases presenting in an unusual way. Doctors are well aware of this, but very few patients have any idea of the scale of the difficulty. Over and above the intrinsic difficulties in diagnosis, it is remarkable how manifold are the sources of error. An editorial in the *British Medical Journal*[7] summed it up well:

> " *The physician may be hurried, impatient, tired,*
> *inexperienced, prejudiced, unsympathetic, or negligent.*
> *The patient may be foolish, timid, aggressive, taciturn,*
> *loquacious, ignorant or untruthful. How often does the*
> *common human frailty of examiner and examined*
> *combine to frustrate the best intentions of both.*"

When the patient has little English or poor hearing, and when he has been directed to the wrong specialist, opportunities for mistakes and misunderstanding are compounded.

Deaf and foreign patients inevitably take longer than normal to deal with. We have all experienced a sensation of 'heart-sink' on having such a patient ushered into our consulting room when we were in a hurry. I have worked with consultants who did not hide their impatience with such patients. We need to put ourselves in the patient's position; after all, we might be in the same situation ourselves one day if we are taken ill on an overseas holiday!

Listening

An appropriate questionnaire, as described in the previous chapter, helps to avoid omissions from the history and to make the dates of events more precise. But the patient comes primarily to be listened to and examined by a doctor he trusts. The importance of listening, and showing the patient you are listening, to his story cannot be exaggerated. However short the time may be, it is important for the doctor to make the patient feel that for that brief period he is giving him his full attention. This applies supremely to difficult consultations in which the patient has sought help unsuccessfully before.

It is important to let the patient talk. The doctor should listen and only ask a question to lead him on. One successful physician[8] said:

> "I obey Osler's dictum: 'Listen to the patient: he is
> telling you the diagnosis.' I never interrupt a patient. I
> take down all that she tells me. I read it back to her
> and I say if she remembers anything I have left out she
> must tell me. So the patient feels I really know her case.
> That ensures her confidence in me".

Unfortunately, doctors have a reputation for impatience and an unwillingness to listen. One patient exclaimed to a surgical friend of mine, with surprised appreciation: "**You actually listened to me!**" Listening, in itself, has a therapeutic effect. This is amusingly illustrated by an example which Dr Martyn Lloyd-Jones[9] gave of a consultation by his former 'chief', Lord Horder. I give the story in Lloyd-Jones' own words.

*"One day, Sir Thomas, later Lord, Horder, physician
to St Bartholomew's Hospital, was asked to see a very
distinguished patient — a duchess. The local
practitioner had written a letter of introduction and
had told him that he was sure that there was nothing
really wrong with her, though she thought there was.
She had been to see most of the distinguished
consultants in Harley Street, as well as on the
Continent. But she felt no better; and someone had
suggested Horder. As it happened, the previous
consultation before the arrival of the duchess, had been
a most interesting medical problem in differential
diagnosis at which Horder excelled. This particular
patient had been misdiagnosed and Horder had
discovered what was really the matter with him, and
could see that he could be cured.*

*On the arrival of the duchess, Horder simply
said: 'Please tell me about your symptoms and
experience. I will ask you a question now and again.
But just take your time and tell me.' So she began.
While she was talking, he was busy writing a letter to
the doctor of the previous patient. Now and again, he
would stop and put a question to her. Then he would
go on writing to the doctor concerned with the
previous case, and the duchess went on speaking. This
continued until he had finished writing the letter to the
previous doctor, giving him the diagnosis, his reasons
for it and the suggested treatment. Then he told the
duchess to go on a bit longer and added: 'Well now,
this is most interesting.' He then proceeded to examine
her chest and to take other steps to exclude the presence
of what might be lurking signs of any serious
condition. At the end of the consultation, she said:
'You know, Sir Thomas, I am sure that you are going
to cure me.' 'Oh,' he said, 'How do you know that?'
She replied: 'You are the first doctor who has taken the
trouble to listen to me'."*

Although Horder was not really listening, he had won the patient's confidence in a way that no-one else had, and he was able to deal successfully with her hypochondria. He was able to help because she received the impression that he was patiently following her explanations.

Listening may be therapeutic even if you do not understand what the patient is saying. A teacher from the Buchan area of northeast Scotland came to a marriage guidance counsellor for help with her marriage. She was very distressed, and spoke in a dialect which her counsellor, who was English, found totally unintelligible. After a long time, the counsellor said: "*Well, I think that is as far as we can go today. Come back and see me again next week.*" In the meantime, the counsellor consulted her superior, told her that she had understood nothing, and suggested that she should pass her case over to someone local. The adviser rejected this suggestion. When the client returned, she thanked the counsellor profusely for her help of the previous week, and said that it had enabled her to see the solution to her problem. She insisted on making a donation to the organisation!

Many doctors are convinced that patients take up too much time describing their complaints, and feel the need for a strategy for cutting them short. It therefore comes as something of a surprise to find that the average patient, when allowed to talk without interruption, does not speak for more than two minutes[10,11].

Occasionally, the consultant is left in doubt as to the real reason for the patient's attendance. The general practitioner's letter may not tell the whole truth. In an analysis of referrals to medical clinics in Edinburgh, Hodge *et al*[12] found that, in a large proportion of cases, the specific indication for referral was unstated, distorted or lost in transmission.

Sometimes, if the disease is chronic and intractable, or if the patient is a hypochondriac, the purpose of referral may be to provide moral support for the family doctor. On other occasions, I have concluded that the patient had been referred because the general practitioner felt that he was under criticism for past neglect, or because of unstated social reasons.

The doctor as detective

Not all that a patient says can be taken at face value. Everybody wants to create a good impression. In particular, patients cannot be trusted to be honest about their drinking and smoking habits. With regard to alcohol consumption, a good suggestion is to ask the patient, "*What is your favourite drink?*" and to follow this up with the question: "*Do you drink a bottle a day?*" The estimate is purposely aimed ridiculously high in order to test the patient's reaction. An immediate dismissal of the idea virtually excludes it, but any hesitation while calculations are made suggests the near accuracy of the statement[13].

Sometimes the main cause of a patient's anxiety is something quite different from what had been suspected. One doctor, when presented with a patient who was obviously unhappy, asked her to write a list of all the things that were troubling her. The doctor went through the list, item by item: her husband had been made redundant; the baby cried a lot at night; a neighbour had said something rude to her over the garden wall and, two weeks previously, the dog had died. It was at this point that the patient's eyes filled with tears, and it became obvious that the death of her dog was her main problem[14].

I have had several similar experiences. One of my patients, a woman in her 60s, wrote to me after a consultation to explain her grief. She told me that she had lost her daughter two years ago, but that the following year she had an even deeper sorrow. She had acquired "*a very dear little squirrel to love and care for.*" He suffered a lingering illness, during which she nursed him for several months. He slept in her room, and during the last weeks of his life, she wrote: "*wee McTavish lived on my person night and day, snuggled in my old cardigan between my left shoulder and my chin.*" When he died, she was plunged into grief, "*trying to hang on to my sanity and keep going with the business of living alone.*"

Sometimes the patient's anxiety about his illness appears totally out of proportion to its severity. There is usually a good reason for this, and one which the doctor needs to deal with thoroughly. A young woman complained persistently of joint pains. There was nothing to see and her complaint appeared greatly exaggerated, until it came out that a close friend of hers had gradually become crippled by rheumatoid arthritis.

At follow-up, it is often very difficult to know whether the patient is feeling better or not. Some patients are reluctant to confess that they are feeling better for fear that the doctor may not re-examine them. Others pretend to feel better than they do, in order to please the doctor and not to appear 'soft'.

Regional differences in symptomatology

There are undoubtedly regional differences in the manner and intensity with which patients present their complaints. I was impressed by this fact when I moved from London to Aberdeen. During the ten years I worked in London, I found that a high proportion of patients gave exaggerated descriptions of their symptoms and many were 'poly-symptomatic'. In a cardiac clinic, many patients complained of pain not only in the front of the chest, but in the side and back and in other remote areas. When I moved up to northeast Scotland, I soon discovered that patients there were more likely to minimise their symptoms than to exaggerate them.

In London, the commonest form of chest pain seen in patients attending the National Heart Hospital was the classic neurotic left inframammary pain: *"It's the heart, doctor"* — said with an anguished expression. In Aberdeen, however, this presentation was quite rare. In London, it was the practice to determine the severity of mitral stenosis mainly on the basis of symptoms, particularly breathlessness, which was graded I–IV. In Aberdeen, I found patients with potentially fatal mitral stenosis who admitted to virtually no breathlessness at all! Later, I was interested to discover that Sir Robert Hutchison, who was brought up in Midlothian, Scotland, but practised in London, had observed the same phenomenon. He used to say[15]:

> *"The value of a history decreases progressively as you go from Banff to Brighton."*

The doctor's questions

The booklet *Talking with Patients* edited by Lord Walton, contains an excellent interviewing model[16]. This suggests that the doctor should start with an entirely open question, such as *"What is your problem?"* Other opening gambits can easily misfire. *"Why have you come to see me?"* is often answered by *"Because my doctor sent me."* *"What is wrong with you?"* invites the reply *"That is what I want you to tell me."*

When the patient dries up, the doctor should ask whether there are any other problems he would like to mention. It is important to ask how much the problem affects the patient and the family. If the patient has majored on organic problems, he should be questioned about changes in mood. This line of enquiry can be continued in a 'cooler' way during the course of physical examination, when the absence of eye contact lowers the tension and encourages the patient to mention sensitive matters in a more casual way. It is important to ask specific questions such as whether the patient has a fear of cancer or heart disease, whether he is depressed, and whether he has contemplated suicide.

When the patient complains of several symptoms, it is valuable to ask him to rank them in order of importance: *"Which is the worst symptom?"*, *"Which is the next worst?"* and finally *"What do you think is the cause of your trouble?"* The patient's idea may be correct or incorrect, but in either case his answer gives a clue to his main fear. The doctor then knows that this is what he must focus on if he is to reassure the patient effectively.

The importance of asking open-ended questions is now widely recognised. The patient may ask the doctor: *"Why do I get these headaches?"* Before attempting to answer, it is often valuable to throw the question back at the patient: *"Why do **you** think you get them?"*

Many patients are impatient over the history taking and are careless about dates, sites of pain, etc. They think they have come to the specialist primarily to be examined. In my experience, this applies particularly to the so-called 'upper classes'. Some patients describe a number of unrelated symptoms without indicating which, if any, interferes with their enjoyment of life.

To avoid breaking the flow with interruptions, no attempt should be made to write down the history in its final form while taking it. I employ a number of abbreviations for rough note-taking. At the end of the history taking, an attempt should be made to list both the most likely and the most serious diagnoses to be considered. In seeking to draw conclusions from a history, the doctor would like to be able to make a single diagnosis which explains everything. This is sometimes possible, but in most cases the best that can be done is to find a diagnosis which explains the most troublesome symptoms. Often, a symptom which appeared at first sight to be significant, proves to be a 'red herring'.

Sometimes the doctor will become aware that the 'physic- al' symptom the patient has presented is only a cover for his real psychological problem. In such a situation, the doctor needs to take the physical complaint seriously. But he also needs to indicate to the patient the need for a proper psychological consultation, either with his general practitioner or with a psychiatric specialist.

Occasionally, the patient is so imprecise, vague and contra-dictory that the history is to all intents and purposes valueless. Sometimes, I have written in my notes: *"Impossible historian!"* In such cases, I try to follow the advice attributed to Dr Charles H Mayo:

> *"When you cannot find out what is wrong with a man who is ill, just ask his wife, and often she will tell you."*

A follower of Dr Mayo added this further advice:

> *"Sometimes, when the man and his wife don't tell you that his family is full of people who are peculiar or 'a bit off', ask a sister-in-law, and she will tell you."*

If no help is forthcoming from relatives, neighbours or business associates, everything depends on the examination.

References

1. Hampton JR, Harrison MJG, Mitchell JRA, Prichard JS, Seymour C (1975) Relative contributions of history taking, physical examination, and laboratory investigation to diagnosis and management of medical outpatients. *Br Med J* **270**: 486–9

2. Simpson M, Buckman R, Stewart M *et al* (1991) Doctor-patient communication: the Toronto consensus statement. *Br Med J* **303**: 1385–7

3. Wilkie A, Wessely S (1994) Patients with medically unexplained symptoms. *Br J Hosp Med* **51**: 421–7

4. Spence J (1953). Function of the hospital out-patient department. *Lancet* **i**: 275

5. Hardy-Roberts GP (1951) Office manners. *Lancet* **i**: 1119-20

6. Tate P (1983) Doctors' style. In Pendleton D, Hasler J, eds. *Doctor-Patient Communication*. Academic Press, London: 79

7. *British Medical Journal* (editorial) (1952) The patient tells his story. *Br Med J* **ii**: 1246–7

8. Howie J (1987). Portraits from memory—Dr Hugh Morton. *Br Med J* **295**: 839–40

9. Lloyd-Jones M (1982) *The Doctor Himself*. Christian Medical Fellowship, London: 44

10. Beckman HB, Frankel RM (1984) The effect of physician behaviour on the collection of data. *Ann Intern Med* **101**: 692–6

11. Blau JN (1989) Time to let the patient speak. *Br Med J* **298**: 39

12. Hodge JAH, Jacob A, Ford MJ, Munro JF (1992) Medical clinic referral letters. Do they say what they mean? Do they mean what they say? *Scott Med J* **37**: 179–80

13. Welsby P (1989) Non-medical practice makes perfect. *Proc R Coll Physicians Edinb*, **19**: 98–9

14. Elliott-Binns CP (1981) Personal View. *Br Med J* **282**: 1230

15. Hunter D (1971) Centenary of the birth of Robert Hutchison. *Br Med J* **263**: 222–3

16. Walton J, ed (1980) *Talking with Patients*. Nuffield Provincial Hospitals Trust, London

Chapter 4
THE SCIENCE AND ART OF DIAGNOSIS

- Physical examination is still essential
- The importance of the psychological dimension
- Computer assistance in diagnosis
- Patient participation in diagnosis
- When diagnosis is not the top priority

It has been claimed, convincingly, that diagnosis is the weakest link in the chain of medical services as they are practised today[1]. This chapter examines the reason for this and considers the potential of the computer to improve the situation.

The logical sequel to history taking is physical examination. However, the scope of such examination varies so much from one specialty to another that it is more useful in a book such as this to focus on principles rather than details of practice. In doing so, I start with a warning.

The danger of neglect of physical examination

There is a danger that, with the passing of the years, the successful doctor will tend to cut corners and omit routine procedures which are usually negative. The reduction in the availability of nurses to act as chaperones may also influence doctors so that they omit 'intimate examinations' such as palpation of the breast, and digital examination of the rectum and vagina. Inevitably, the specialist also tends to become 'rusty' in the recognition and treatment of diseases outside his own specialty. Fortunately, patients admitted to state hospitals are examined by junior doctors who, although lacking experience, still retain a broad knowledge of disease and are likely to follow the routine they have been taught. However, as this safeguard does not always exist in the case of patients admitted to private hospitals, it is important that consultants should attend regular refresher courses which include recent advances in specialties other than their own. It seems likely that this will soon become compulsory.

Doctors should always explain the examinations they wish to undertake, and give appropriate reassurance. This is particularly important when the patient comes from another culture and when the examination involves the perineum or the breasts. If the patient's comprehension of the English language is poor, it may be necessary to enlist the help of an interpreter.

Another danger is that, with the steadily increasing availability of investigations, clinical examination will be regarded as superfluous and, as a result, skills will atrophy. Indeed, there is evidence that this is already happening in paediatric medicine[2] and in cardiac auscultation[3]. Some years ago, while on a visit to a prestigious centre abroad, I was shown a patient with a cardiac murmur in whom extensive investigations, some of them invasive, had failed to elucidate the diagnosis. Careful bedside examination showed that the patient had a mild mitral valve lesion for which no sophisticated investigations were necessary.

If every patient was investigated by advanced technology, the health service would be overwhelmed and costs would escalate. Moreover, the patient would suffer because most investigations are uncomfortable, carry occasional risks and, from time to time, throw up anomalous and misleading results which require further investigation. Hampton[4] has put it well in saying:

> *"Intelligent use of scarce and expensive investigational technology depends on a good history and an accurate physical examination."*

Goodwin[5] has emphasised that the more complex high technology becomes, the more basic skills are needed and the more difficult it will be to restore them once they are lost. In any case, there are situations in which a doctor has to examine a patient in circumstances where no technology is available, for example, on a domiciliary visit. Apart from the evidence it elicits, physical examination is an impressive and powerful ritual[6], which strengthens the bond between doctor and patient.

Failure to appreciate the psychological dimension

A third danger is that of concentrating on physical signs to the exclusion of the psychological component of the patient's symptoms. It is all too easy to find an abnormal sign and make it carry the full weight of responsibility for the patient's illness. Balint[7] has emphasised this danger, saying:

"It is a mistake to regard physical illness as always more important than functional illness ... There is a danger, not only in missing a physical sign but in finding one."

He warned against allowing a patient to 'organise' his illness round an unimportant physical finding, such as extra systoles, a heart murmur, mild hypertension or a hiatus hernia.

An acute emotional disturbance unwisely handled may lead to chronic invalidism. For example, a fright may cause unpleasant palpitation and raise a suspicion of heart disease. If this is handled imprudently, and the patient is told about an innocent cardiac murmur and advised to rest, he may become a cardiac cripple.

Complaints of persistent exhaustion and tiredness are often psychogenic. A 50-year-old woman complained of exhaustion, palpitation and dyspnoea, but questioning elicited the information that she had no symptoms when playing golf or curling. It was revealed later that her mother was living with her, and the patient could see no end to this burden. A 60-year-old male surgeon complained of exhaustion, which persisted in spite of a good holiday on one of the Greek islands. There was no evidence of any disease, and it transpired that he was current chairman of his specialty division and was engaged in a difficult and unpleasant battle with his administrative superior.

Computer assistance in diagnosis

The concept of computer assistance in diagnosis is attractive and logical, and it is surprising that it is not more widely used. As long ago as 1972, De Dombal[8] demonstrated its value in the diagnosis of abdominal pain. This has since been abundantly confirmed, as has its value in the diagnosis of chest pain[9].

The computer offers a list of possible diagnoses too large to be handled by most human brains, together with probability estimates for each disease. It can also act as a safeguard against common errors, and a check against the tendency to be over-influenced by one's most recent experience.

The question may be asked: why merely computer assistance? Why not computer diagnosis? A fully computerised diagnostic service is indeed conceivable, and is available in principle, but there are various reasons why it is inappropriate for the foreseeable future[1]. The chief reason is that information provided by the computer is not infallible. There are several reasons for this. In the first place, its programming can never be fully comprehensive and up to date. It reflects established specialist knowledge rather than the latest advances. Moreover, it is forced to ignore rare cases. Every patient's complaint is unique or at least contains a unique component, and this cannot be handled by the computer.

Although the computer cannot safely be allowed to make the diagnosis, it can undoubtedly help by suggesting diagnoses which the doctor might otherwise overlook. Moreover, its value is not confined to the first consultation but continues throughout the period of observation. The response to treatment, and future developments, can be fed into it and yield fresh ideas.

Computer-mediated on-line searching of the biomedical literature can also provide valuable assistance in acute medical care[10]. The computer may also be able to give an estimate of prognosis, and thus help in decisions about the withdrawal of intensive therapy.

The fact that computer assistance has not been more enthusiastically embraced by physicians is partly due to the development of the hospital information support system project towards an administrative rather than a clinical application[11]. It also reflects a fear that computerisation would be a further step in the direction of depersonalised medicine. In fact, the opposite should be the case. The computer should set the physician free to do what a physician can do best, namely to concentrate on the patient's individual and unique needs[12].

Patient participation in diagnosis

An important potential application of the computer is to encourage the patient to participate more fully in the diagnostic and decision-making processes. For a start, the patient could use the computer to help him decide whether it was necessary to consult a doctor, thereby replacing popular encyclopaedias and handbooks of medicine. The patient's use of the computer in the process of consultation would ensure his informed consent. Patients would be given a standard set of explanations and then be invited to decide their input into the diagnostic process. In so doing, they would soon come to realise the importance of an accurate history and also that concealing or giving misleading information would lead to an unreliable diagnosis.

When it comes to a decision regarding further investigation and treatment, the use of a computer would increase the patient's options. Patients vary greatly in the weight they attach to the risks of investigations and treatment. In carcinoma of the breast, for instance, the value that women attach to retention of the breast over and against the risk of recurrence and death varies widely. The goal of computer assistance would be to establish the patient as the decision maker at all stages in diagnosis and treatment.

When precise diagnosis is not the top priority

It is a mistake to regard diagnosis as an end in itself. Diagnosis is simply a key step towards appropriate management. Decisions regarding treatment should be guided more by prognosis than by diagnosis. Thus, it is often prudent to act on a less likely diagnosis when the consequence of therapeutic neglect would be serious. For example, in a patient with abdominal pain, laparotomy may be indicated even if the probability of appendicitis is lower than that of non-specific pain. There is a need for more research to be undertaken to discover the likely outcomes of different treatments, with the aim of updating our knowledge base and guiding future decision-making[13].

A precise diagnosis should not be pursued if it cannot lead to any improvement in the patient's condition. Too often, sick people are subjected to physical and mental suffering in the course of investigations that are a waste of time and money. For a patient who is old or frail or just ill, any trip to the X-ray department, even for a simple plain radiograph, can be a trial. We need to keep in mind Hutchison's litany[14]:

> *"From inability to leave well alone;*
> *From too much zeal for the new and contempt for*
> *what is old;*
> *From putting knowledge before wisdom, science before*
> *art, and cleverness before common sense,*
> *From treating patients as cases, and from making the*
> *cure of the disease more grievous than the endurance of*
> *the same,*
> *Good Lord, deliver us. "*

Of course, this advice must not be made an excuse for mental laziness, or for writing off patients who might be cured. The pursuit of a diagnosis should always have as its goal the patient's benefit rather than the doctor's intellectual satisfaction.

References

1.   Laor N, Agassi J (1990) *Diagnosis: Philosophical and Medical Perspectives*. Kluwer Academic Publishers, Dordrecht

2. Macadessi J, Oates RK (1993) Clinical diagnosis of pyloric stenosis: a declining art. *Br Med J* **306**: 553–5

3. Mangione S, Nieman LZ, Gracely E, Kaye D (1993) The teaching and practice of cardiac auscultation during internal medicine and cardiology training. *Arch Intern Med* **119**: 47–54

4. Hampton JR (1993) Book review. *Br Med J* **306**: 595

5. Goodwin J (1995) The importance of clinical skills. *Br Med J* **310**: 1281–2

6. Tate P (1983) Doctors' style. In: Pendleton D, Hasler J, eds. *Doctor—Patient Communication*. Academic Press, London: 81

7. Balint M (1964). *The Doctor, His Patient and the Illness*. Pitman, London: 62

8. De Dombal FT (1972) Computer aided diagnosis of acute abdominal pain. *Br Med J* **265**: 9–13

9. Wyatt J (1991) Computer-based knowledge systems. *Lancet* **338**: 1431–6

10. Lindberg DAB, Siegel ER, Rapp BA, Wallingford KT, Wilson SR (1993) Computer-mediated searching of the biomedical literature. *JAMA* **269**: 3124–9

11. Lelliott P (1994) Making clinical informatics work. *Br Med J* **308**: 802–3

12. Peset JL, Gracia D (1992) *The ethics of diagnosis*. Kluwer Academic Publishers, Dordrecht

13. Delamothe T (1994) Using outcomes research in clinical practice. *Br Med J* **308**: 1583–4

14. Hutchison R (1953) Modern treatment (letter). *Br Med J* **226**: 671

Chapter 5
PRINCIPLES OF PATIENT MANAGEMENT

◆ The importance of an actual diagnosis
◆ Reassurance
◆ Honesty
◆ Don't be a spoilsport
◆ Paternalism
◆ 'Decision analysis'
◆ Rehabilitation
◆ Planning investigations
◆ Follow-up
◆ Supporting the general practitioner

Once the doctor has taken the history and completed his examination, the patient expects a diagnosis and advice.

An actual diagnosis is important. It conveys the feeling that the doctor knows what is wrong, and it rules out other dreaded possibilities which may have been in the patient's mind. A retired physician, Dr Grant, told me that he consulted the professor of orthopaedics about a severe pain in his wrist. The professor did not know the diagnosis, but recommended the use of a splint for a week. This did no good, so he put the forearm in plaster. This gave complete and permanent relief. Three months later, the surgeon was consulted by a lady with a similar story. He told her the condition wasn't serious and that a week in plaster would put it right. The patient asked what the diagnosis was; the surgeon replied that it was a rare but curable condition. The patient thought he was concealing something, and insisted on a name for the disease. Under pressure, the surgeon said: *"Well, it's called Grant's syndrome."* This satisfied her. A few weeks later, she was in London for a family wedding. There she met a doctor friend and told him about her experience and the diagnosis she had been given. *"Grant's* syndrome?", he said, *"I've never heard of it."*

At an early stage, it may not be possible to give a positive diagnosis. Further investigations may be necessary. Balint[1] (whose advice to general practitioners is equally applicable to specialists) warned against advising or reassuring the patient until the doctor is sure what the real problem is. Nevertheless, it may be possible to offer some limited reassurance. For example, the doctor may be in a position to say *"The complete picture is not yet clear, but you'll be glad to hear that your heart is all right."* or *"There's no sign of cancer."*

Reassurance

The importance of truthful reassurance and encouragement cannot be exaggerated. All clinical teachers of experience are agreed on this. Dr William Evans (who was famous for his aphorisms on patient management) used to say:

> *" Among the many medicaments which doctors carry in their bags, there can be none more precious than reassurance: precious in that it is the 'pill' he has to dispense most frequently, and so often does most good."*

Unfortunately, doctors are not as good at this as they should be, so that what Dr George Day[2] said many years ago is still true:

> *"There is an enormous amount of ill-health and wasted life all around us, simply because patients and ex-patients are not relieved of their uncertainty."*

The need for reassurance may not be as great in psychotherapy, concerning which Balint[1] has said that when the doctor and patient diagnose the problem, there is usually no need for formal advice and reassurance, and no value in these exercises. But it is certainly true in the case of physical illness. Kessel[3] advised:

> *"The uttering of reassurance should be as planned and*

deliberate as the use of any other medical skill."

Reassurance is often most effective if it is indirect. One good method of indirect reassurance is for the doctor in charge to explain the situation to a junior doctor, student or nurse in the presence of the patient, in simple terms which the patient can understand, and then repeat it to the patient[4]. Another method, which I have sometimes used, is to close a consultation with a patient who has a bad prognosis with the request: *"Send me a postcard in a year's time and let me know how you are getting on."*

Reassurance should, if possible, be unqualified. So often the doctor's reassurance is unnecessarily guarded: *"You have done well but don't go out by yourself."* Or to a patient who has had a heart attack: *"You'll be all right now, provided you don't get another attack"* or *"Yes, of course you may play golf, but don't walk up inclines"*. Unless the qualification is essential, it should be omitted because it tends to sow seeds of doubt in the patient's mind. Most would agree that it is better to enjoy life to the full for a short time than to eke out a miserable and apprehensive existence for a few more years.

Reassurance should be prompt. Patients are often kept anxiously waiting for the results of tests long after they have been reported. In this context, no news is certainly not good news. Doctors should use the telephone more, asking the patient to phone in as soon as convenient after the time at which the results can reasonably be expected.

Some patients need repeated reassurance. This applies particularly to conditions such as cancer and coronary heart disease, which the patient knows are likely to recur. In the case of cancer, reassurance often involves repeated X-rays or other expensive and potentially unpleasant investigations. In the case of coronary disease, it usually necessitates repeated full electro-cardiograms. When serious organic disease is associated with chronic anxiety, the doctor has a difficult long-term problem on his hands.

Some patients are virtually impervious to reassurance. I had such a patient, a doctor's widow, with coronary heart disease. Almost every time I saw her I had not only to repeat her electrocardiogram, but also to demonstrate it to her and show her that there was no deterioration by comparison with the previous tracing. After I had seen her many times, she gave me a clue to her attitude. She told me that her husband used to boast to her of the way he deceived his patients. She thought all doctors were like that.

Sometimes, by a sort of sixth sense, or pronoia, the doctor suspects that the patient has a worry or fear to which he has not admitted. Often, it is cancer or heart disease. He should then, almost casually, scotch this fear in the course of his explanation. Spence[5] gives an excellent example of this. A mother came to see him with her mentally defective baby. He sensed that the mother felt guilty that she had caused the trouble by something she did during her pregnancy. So, in the course of his explanation to the mother, he included a specific reassurance that the child's condition was no fault of hers.

Honesty

Honesty is a fundamental principle of the doctor/patient relationship. The doctor should not deceive his patient, and the patient should be able to trust his doctor to present the situation and answer his questions truthfully. As Joseph Fletcher[6] put it:

> *"The patient has 'opened his books' to the doctor on the reasonable assumption that what is found there will be turned over to him."*

This does not mean that the whole truth has to be imparted right away. Discouraging facts should not be forced upon a patient who does not ask for them.

In this connection, it is important to bear two points in mind. The first is that in medical practice, the relevant facts are rarely known with absolute certainty. In particular, the prognosis is never known precisely. I have often found that my expectations have been far too gloomy. Early in my consultant career, I was called at 5.30 a.m. to see a man of 49 who had just sustained a massive myocardial infarction. On my return home I told my wife that I did not think he would survive the day. In fact he lived a very active life for another 24 years, dying at the age of 73. Not long after, I saw a woman of 51 with severe heart disease, and electrocardiographic features which, according to established teaching, indicated a survival of less than three years. This patient is alive and well a quarter of a century later. If either spouse had asked me "*What do you honestly think about the outlook?*", I would have given a gloomy forecast. And I would have been wrong. So the lesson is that the doctor should have a bias towards optimism. He should never extinguish hope.

Even if the news is bad, it is almost always possible to soften it and impart it gently. Simple gestures of kindness and encouragement go a long way. In cardiological practice, I found myself not infrequently having to advise surgery to someone who dreaded operation, sometimes because they knew a relative who had died after one. I found that a successful way of broaching the subject, if the need for surgery was definite but not urgent, was to say to the patient:

> "*Of course you do not need an operation now. Carry on with medical treatment and come to see me again in two or three months time.*"

I almost invariably found that it was not long before the patient was saying:

> "*What about that operation you mentioned last time? Do you think I ought to have it soon?*"

And a few months later:

> "*How long would I have to wait for the operation? I'd like to get on with it.*"

There are some diagnoses which patients, in their ignorance, regard as a death sentence. I was checking up an 80-year-old woman for possible anaemia, and received a haematological report of leukaemia. I knew very well that the old lady was an inveterate worrier, and I saw no point in troubling her with a diagnosis which would inevitably have alarmed her, for which I could have provided no convincing reassurance and, moreover, which required no treatment. She eventually died at the age of 92 from a hypertensive stroke, unaware of the leukaemia, which had caused her no trouble.

The other point to bear in mind is that when a patient does not ask for clarification about his diagnosis and prognosis, it is often because he believes that the news will be bad, and does not want this confirmed. He would sooner live with an element of doubt and a glimmer of hope, than in hopeless certainty.

A friend of mine said to her consultant, after the results of her investigations had all come in: *"Doctor, I want you to tell me exactly what is wrong with me."* The doctor looked her straight in the face and said: *"Do you really want to know?"* The patient paused for a moment and said: *"Well, no."* The specialist concluded by saying that he would ask her general practitioner to come and talk things over with her. The patient accepted that.

In imparting information to patients with cancer, a valuable way of conducting a gradual enlightenment is to ask at each stage: *"What have they told you so far?"* The exception to this rule of gradual enlightenment is when the doctor has reason to believe that the patient needs to know the full facts, without delay, in order to make an appropriate decision regarding treatment and provision for the future.

In the past, it was the practice to inform the patient's next of kin of a serious diagnosis before informing the patient. Often, indeed, the patient was never told the diagnosis by the doctor. This seems still to be the practice in some quarters. It is, of course, mistaken, as a rule, and the General Medical Council's 'blue book' makes it clear that such unauthorised disclosure should occur only in exceptional circumstances[7].

The question arises as to whether the doctor should warn the patient about all the possible mishaps and side-effects of treatment or only the commonest ones. The patient is, of course, entitled to know everything, and should be told everything if he requests it. Most patients, however, have come to the specialist for advice and are satisfied to accept his suggestion, and consider any options he offers. In my view, it depends on how essential the proposed treatment is. If the treatment has to be gone through in any case, the less fear and anxiety surrounding it the better. Everyone knows that there are risks attached to any operation. When I underwent my hip replacement, it would not have helped me to know that I might suffer a fatal pulmonary embolism, or permanent liver or brain damage from the anaesthetic. Similarly, in the case of essential chemotherapy, side-effects are to be expected, and the patient must be warned about them. However, the warning should be in general terms, because the side-effects are diverse and individualistic, and there is a danger of making them worse by focusing the patient's attention on them.

Don't be a spoilsport

The doctor should never spoil a patient's enjoyment of life without some very compelling reason. Too many doctors put their patients on drugs or diets without any definite proof that they do any good. For example, consider the matter of dietary advice for the avoidance of coronary heart disease. For years, the entire English-speaking world was urged to avoid butter and cut down on dairy products, in spite of the fact that its value was never proven. I am glad to be able to look back over nearly a quarter of a century of consulting practice and say that I never advised any of my patients to renounce butter. Friends who invited me for a meal would often get in a fresh supply of a butter-substitute "for the doctor". But they were left to dispose of it themselves!

Many doctors spoil their patients' lives by telling them about unimportant and irrelevant signs such as murmurs and extrasystoles, of which they are unaware. Such useless information tends to lead to what Dr William Evans used to call 'unwarranted cardiac invalidism'.

In the past, many patients were subjected to unnecessary operations — dental extractions to eradicate septic foci, colectomy for visceroptosis, prophylactic circumcision, sympathectomy for hypertension and for Raynaud's disease—the list is endless. There can be no doubt that doctors are still undertaking unnecessary surgery. Not so long ago, operations for tonsillectomy, haemorrhoidectomy and inguinal herniorhaphy were performed twice as frequently in North America as in the UK, and cholecystectomy rates were five times greater. Hysterectomy rates in the USA were eight times as high as those in Norway[8]. Perhaps this tendency is greater where surgeons are paid on an item of service basis. At all events, there is undoubtedly a tremendous amount of iatrogenic illness, and every doctor should take pains to avoid adding to it. We should remember Dr William Evans' first maxim: *"No patient should be the worse for seeing a doctor."*

Sometimes the doctor finds himself in an acutely difficult position in trying to avoid being a spoilsport as, for example, when a patient is taken ill shortly before a long-awaited and expensive holiday. The hardest decision I ever had to make was when a retired senior colleague with coronary heart disease had a fresh attack of anginal pain at rest on the eve of a world tour. His electrocardiogram showed obvious deterioration. The patient was of a nervous disposition, and the pain had subsided by the time I saw him. He wanted to go provided that it was not foolhardy. He was a widower. I decided not to advise against going, but told him to avoid exertion as far as possible for a week or two. I also confided in a mutual friend and colleague, who agreed with my decision. The patient returned safely from the experience of a lifetime.

Paternalism

Doctors are widely criticised for being too paternalistic, and there is no doubt a large measure of truth in the accusation. Indeed, we are more paternalistic than we often realise. Most of us think nothing of withholding information, telling the patient half-truths, imparting so-called 'health education' — all for the patient's good, of course! Increasingly, 'professional dominance' is resented and 'patient power' is sought. But if it true that 'knowledge is power', then professional dominance is inevitable in a doctor/patient relationship. Furthermore, this seems to be what most patients want in practice.

Most patients look for an element of direction from their medical advisers. For example, a study of 150 women with recently diagnosed breast cancer showed that only 20% wanted an active role in deciding their treatment; 28% preferred to share decision making, and 52% wished the surgeon to decide[9]. In my experience, this desire for the decision to be made by the consultant is true of most doctors when they become patients.

There is also considerable evidence, at least in general practice, that a 'directing' form of consultation is more effective than a 'sharing' one[10]. It seems that an egalitarian therapeutic relationship diminishes the doctor's magical healing and anxiety-relieving power[11]. Faith in the doctor is an important ingredient in cure.

As a general principle, I believe that patients should be given the essential facts and the treatment options, and then be invited to make their own choice. For this, they need the fullest and most accurate information available to the doctor. In future, this process may be facilitated by the use of an interactive video system, as described in an earlier chapter. This could be programmed with the most up-to-date information, and lead the patient step by step to his own decision. The outcome of treatment in each case could later be fed into the system to update the information for future users.

There can be no doubt that doctors are finding their patients increasingly well informed on all medical issues, and increasingly prepared to dispute the doctor's recommendations. Inevitably, some intelligent patients are going to be better informed than their medical adviser regarding their own illness. Often, however, the patient's understanding is flawed, or his information is unconfirmed or out of date, and it rarely takes account of the individual patient's idiosyncrasies.

In advocating a degree of paternalism, I am far from suggesting that a doctor should foist his views on his patients. This applies particularly to situations such as requests for termination of pregnancy, on which there are strongly held differences of opinion.

The doctor may be opposed to such action in principle, but his duty is to help his patient to a wise decision within the parameters of his or her own philosophy of life.

The doctor should also take care to prevent the patient becoming dependent on him. It is a laudable objective to make the patient, as far as possible, his own physician.

Decision analysis

Reaching a wise decision may be aided by decision analysis. This is a method for breaking down complex problems of management into their component parts, analysing the parts in detail, and then combining them in a logical way to indicate the best course of action[12]. Decision analysis is based on a comprehensive survey of the world literature, supplemented by experience locally regarding the outcome of various treatment regimen. It replaces the tendency for doctors to decide by intuition or on the basis of personal experience, which is often biased by the most recent success or failure. It is now recognised[13] that clinical information systems have an important role in the delivery of 'evidence-based clinical practice'.

Wrong decisions are made partly as a result of well-recognised biases, and partly because of a failure to recognise the range of patients' values and weigh them correctly. Decision analysis is designed to take account of the patient's preferences. In carcinoma of the breast, for instance, the patient can indicate her weighting of the risk of recurrence and death versus retention of the breast. In carcinoma of the cervix, she can indicate the value she places on the retention of fertility over and against an increased risk of death.

Decision analysis is seldom used in its full rigour for the treatment of individual patients. More often, it helps to structure debate on treatment in general in the case of such controversies as the management of appendicitis, antibiotic treatment for sore throats, coronary artery bypass surgery, and the management of intracranial aneurysms. It is a means to the goal of appropriate care, that is treatment in which the benefits can be expected to exceed the risks by a wide enough margin to make it worth providing[14]. Ignorance, incompetence, poor management and sometimes deliberate disregard of established knowledge all militate against appropriate care[15].

Rehabilitation

A good doctor wants to see his patient not only diagnosed and treated, but also rehabilitated. Changes in the patient's life-style need to be discussed with him if they are to be effective, and the advice should be specific. In the case of a patient who has suffered a heart attack causing permanent limitation of physical strength, it is no good advising a reduction in activities in vague and general terms, such as: *"You should cut down on your work load"* or *"You should take more rest".* The advice must be precise: *"You should keep the weekend free"* and, if the situation warrants it, *"I would strongly suggest that you take a day off in the middle of the week as well."*

In such cases, I made it my practice to ask the patient to make a list of his commitments in order of importance, putting at the top those which are of the greatest interest to him and which only he can do, and ending with those which do not really interest him and might equally well be done by others. Then I suggested that he should draw a line halfway down and take immediate steps to shed the lower half. I would point out that he would never have a better chance of cutting down his workload. News of his illness was bound to evoke sympathy and cooperation, especially if backed by 'doctor's orders'. I am, of course, speaking of situations in which the patient's wellbeing requires a reduction in workload. There are patients who are physically fit, but who use illness as an opportunity for what Balint described as *"withdrawal from all sorts of unsatisfactory or frustrating, demanding or over-exacting relationships with other people"*[1].

Sometimes, the process of rehabilitation is difficult and time-consuming, particularly in patients with long-standing illness. Although this is more the province of the general practitioner than of the specialist, the specialist may be able to play a crucial role. There is a remarkable example of such action in the biography of Lord Dawson. His course of action was admittedly exceptional and indeed daring, but it is a good illustration of the lengths to which a specialist should be prepared to go if he is to do his best for his patient.

Lord Dawson's patient was interested in public life and had parliamentary aspirations. He had developed an intestinal neurosis and used to take a diet with him to dinner parties. He spent much time thinking of and discussing his abdominal feelings. Dawson gave him a cold-blooded analysis of his disease, pointing out that it must have started with some kind of intestinal upset and this had led to the neurosis with increasing egoism and decreasing interest in others. He pointed out that he was well on the way towards ruining his public career. He advised him that he was going to make a public diagnosis of long-standing appendix trouble and advise that he should have the appendix operated on. This would justify and explain his conduct in the eyes of the public. The patient was to stick to this explanation and say absolutely nothing else to any other person except his wife. On the other hand, he was to understand that the operation would only be the first chapter of his treatment and that he would require six to eight weeks under medical care in the country to train his intestine back into rational tolerance, to train his abdomen back into unconsciousness, and to train his mind to forget himself. It is related that the patient recovered his health and spirits and went on to an active public career[16].

Before ending a consultation, the doctor should never lose any opportunity for health promotion. Smoking should be strongly discouraged, advice should be given on weight reduction and exercise, where appropriate, and evidence of an unhealthy lifestyle should be brought pointedly to the patient's attention.

Planning investigations

In planning further investigations, the doctor must take care to avoid exhausting the patient. This result is, alas, all too common in hospital, because of a laudable attempt to reach a diagnosis as quickly as possible. In general, it is a good rule to follow 'the line of least annoyance'. Hippocrates said in relation to treatment: *"If the patient can be made well in many ways, choose the least troublesome."* Similarly in relation to investigation, if the diagnosis can be established in many ways, start with the least distressing. Patients should be warned of the side-effects of their investigations.

Many patients become unnecessarily alarmed about tests such as intravenous pyelograms and scans, which doctors readily order for patients without any explanation. They should be told why each test is needed, what it involves, and whether it will be painful. Some patients, especially the youngest ones, find double-contrast barium enemas extremely painful[17]. A proportion of patients undergoing magnetic resonance imaging become acutely anxious and claustrophobic[18].

If, after all appropriate investigations have been done, no relevant disease has been discovered, it is important not to jump to the conclusion that the symptom is imaginary or exaggerated. It is usually best to explain to the patient that the tests have not shown up any significant disease, give appropriate reassurance and indicate that, if the symptoms persist, they would need to be re-investigated. Not infrequently, investigations which show no abnormality at an early stage in the disease do so later. When I suffered a breakdown of my artificial hip after 17 years of use, the first X-ray was reported as showing no abnormality, and I was reassured that there was no evidence of a structural problem. Repeat X-ray three months later showed an obvious fracture of the stem.

The option of seeking the opinion of another specialist is considered in chapter 9.

Follow-up

The question arises as to when the specialist should follow up the patient instead of handing him back directly to the referring doctor. Any follow-up has, of course, to be approved by the general practitioner, and should not be undertaken without very good reason, such as the need to clarify the diagnosis. The main reason for continued hospital surveillance should be that the latest advances in the specialty are not sufficiently familiar to the general practitioner. Other valid reasons for follow-up are the interest and education of the specialist and teaching, but these should be subservient to the welfare of the patient.

In many centres, the hospital outpatient workload is increasing, not because more patients are being referred, but because more patients are being retained. This tendency needs to be strictly limited, and only undertaken with the informed consent of the patient and his general practitioner. Junior staff need instruction in this area of management because they, naturally, have less confidence in discharging patients from follow-up.

Supporting the general practitioner

It is important for the specialist to support the general practitioner, who has the responsibility for the continuing care of the patient. The specialist is simply an expert adviser. He must therefore do nothing to undermine and everything to sustain the patient's confidence in his personal doctor. Although the specialist's advice naturally carries great weight, decisions regarding treatment should, as a general rule, be taken by the patient in conjunction with his general practitioner. This applies particularly to decisions regarding surgery.

Conclusion

Perhaps the most important point on which to conclude this chapter is the need to treat our patients as people. Many doctors who have been patients have complained of a serious lack of communication, particularly when going through operations. One wrote of the fear and loneliness he felt as a surgical patient, in the hands of his colleagues. Another wrote[19]:

> "The operation was never discussed with me... My
> survival has been dependent on the scientific skills of
> many; but curiously enough my best memories are of
> the sympathetic art of a few."

A close friend of mine, who had been through a long illness with many hospital admissions, confided in me that he had found doctors superb in a crisis, but less helpful in day-to-day management.

Patient satisfaction is important. The degree to which the patient feels satisfied with the consultation is strongly associated with the probability that he will comply with advice. Patient compliance is erratic at the best of times, and it is worse if the patient has not understood what is wrong with him and why he needs to take the treatment that has been prescribed. There is evidence that the patient is more likely to follow advice if the doctor is seen as friendly and spends some time in discussion of non-medical topics, rather than being merely businesslike[20].

References

1.   Balint M (1964) The Doctor, His Patient and the Illness. Pitman, London: 260

2.   Day GH (1964) Iatrogenic health. Br Med J i: 1104–7

3.   Kessel N (1979) Reassurance. Lancet 313: 1128–33

4.   Apley J (1980) Communicating with children. Br Med J 281: 1116–7

5. Spence J (1960) *The Purpose and Practice of Medicine*. Oxford University Press, London: 276

6. Fletcher J (1955) *Morals and Medicine*. Gollancz, London: 56

7. General Medical Council (1992) *Professional Conduct and Discipline: Fitness to Practice*. GMC, London: 26–7

8. Andersen TF, Mooney G, eds (1990) *The Challenges of Medical Practice Variations*. Macmillan Press, London

9. Fallowfield LJ, Hall A, Maguire P, Baum M, A'Hern RP (1994) Psychological effects of being offered choice of surgery for breast cancer. *Br Med J* 309: 448

10. Savage R, Armstrong D (1990) Effect of a general practitioner's consulting style on patients' satisfaction: a controlled study. *Br Med J* 301: 968–70

11. Karasu T (1981) Ethical aspects of psychotherapy. In: Bloch S, Chodoff P, eds. *Psychiatric Ethics*. Oxford University Press, Oxford: 98

12. Thornton JG, Lilford RJ, Jonson A (1992) Decision analysis in medicine. *Br Med J* 304: 1099–1103

13. Coiera E (1995) Medical informatics. *Br Med J* 310: 1381–7

14 Brook RH (1994) Appropriateness: the next frontier *Br Med J* 308: 218–19

15. Delamothe T (1993) Wanted: guidelines that doctors will follow. *Br Med J* 307: 218

16. Watson F (1951) *Lord Dawson of Penn*. Chatto and Windus, London: 123

17. Steine S (1993) Will it hurt, doctor? Factors predicting patients' experience of pain during double contrast examination of the colon. *Br Med J* 307: 100

18. Melandez JC, McCrank E (1993) Anxiety-related reactions associated with magnetic resonance imaging examinations. *JAMA* 270: 745–7

19. Green R, ed (1972) *Sick Doctors*. Heinemann, London.

20. Ley P (1977) Patient compliance — a psychologist's viewpoint. *Prescribers J* 17: 15–20

Chapter 6
THE IMPORTANCE OF WORDS

"How good is a timely word." (Proverbs 15;23)

◆ The need for explanation
◆ Answering the patient's questions
◆ Aids to communication
◆ What to avoid

The consultant's top priority is, of course, correct diagnosis and treatment. But, to the patient, communication rates equally highly. Lack of communication is still the commonest complaint which patients level against doctors. How often we still hear the words: *"They never tell you anything."* It is not only the impression the doctor makes and the advice he gives which are important; the actual words he uses are also important. Patients often claim to remember exactly what the doctor said long after the doctor himself has forgotten it — if indeed he ever did utter it! A country general practitioner put it well when he said:

> *"The greatest art, if art there be left in medicine, is to know how to explain simply and truthfully an illness, to assure a patient what can be done for it, to calm their fears and to put ease into dis-ease."*

William Evans used to say:

> *"Doctors should talk more to their patients. Very often words are better therapeutic agents than medicines."*

The importance of explanation

Of course, it is not true that doctors never tell patients anything. Doctors do usually tell patients something. But it must be admitted that we are, on the whole, not good at communicating with our patients. Even when we try to do our best, patients find our explanations inadequate or unintelligible.

Many doctors fail to appreciate the importance of explanation as an ingredient of reassurance. If a patient comes complaining of pain in the chest, it is not sufficient to say: *"There is nothing wrong with your heart or lungs."* The patient wants to know what is causing the pain. In these circumstances, a doctor of my acquaintance used to get the patient to clench his fist or his jaw tightly, to demonstrate to him that contraction of skeletal muscles can be painful. The patient invariably got the point. The idea that some cases of non-cardiac chest pain may be due to unconscious contraction of the chest muscles is supported by the fact that such chest pain is frequently associated with other symptoms consistent with muscular contraction, such as tension headache, tightness in the neck and aching in the shoulders.

Failure to convince a patient that his symptom has no serious basis may lead to chronic invalidism. A patient who had been diagnosed as having advanced cardiac disease was brought into my consulting room in a wheelchair. She had sustained a coronary heart attack a year or so earlier, and ever since had been prone to attacks of chest pain. Many of these occurred at night and necessitated an urgent visit from the doctor. The character of the pain was not unequivocally cardiac, and I found no evidence of deterioration on the electrocardiogram. In these circumstances, it is not possible to be absolutely sure that the symptom is benign, but the situation had become so intolerable that I felt it was worth taking a risk. If I had told the patient that the pain did not arise from her heart, without giving her an alternative explanation, she would have remained unconvinced. I arranged for an X-ray of her chest, and noticed that there was evidence of spondylosis — a common, and usually insignificant, finding. I told her that she had chronic disease of her spine, which wasn't serious, but was the cause of her attacks of pain. She accepted the explanation, and when I saw her again six months later she was walking two miles a day and had never again called her doctor during the night.

Some patients want an explanation for everything but do not have the capacity to understand it. For such patients, Oliver Wendell Holmes[1] advised that the doctor should have a few well-rehearsed phrases always at hand. He added:

> *"As far as possible, keep your doubts to yourself and*
> *give the patient the benefit of your decision."*

As indicated in the previous chapter, there is evidence that in patients in whom no definite diagnosis can be made, a 'positive consultation' — in which a definite diagnosis is given — leads to greater patient satisfaction and a higher recovery rate than a 'negative consultation'.

Patients are rightly annoyed when they receive conflicting information from different members of the team. It is therefore important that key information should, as far as possible, be constantly updated and available to all concerned with patient care.

One of the great problems of communication is that, under the stress of the consultation, patients forget a great deal of what the doctor tells them. In one study it was found that, overall, 40–50% of patients forgot information given them by the doctor[2]. This seems to be particularly true of discouraging or unacceptable information. Patients also frequently misunderstand instructions and reassurance. There is no conclusive evidence as to whether patients remember best what they have been told first or last.

I have already emphasised the importance of reassurance. I would simply add here that the actual words the doctor uses may have a magical effect. A young woman with multiple sclerosis who was referred to a neurologist told him that she had been warned that it might be inadvisable for her to have children. The specialist reassured her with the dramatic words: *"You will have children and grandchildren".*[3]

The fundamental need is for the doctor to appreciate the importance of communication. He owes it to the patient if he is to maximise the effectiveness of his treatment. And he will save himself a lot of trouble if, for any reason, things go wrong. It has been shown that quality of care alone is not an adequate protection against malpractice suits. Breakdown in communication is far more likely to lead to patient dissatisfaction and litigation[4].

Answering the patient's questions

Doctors should ask patients what they want to know and encourage them to ask questions. In answering a patient's questions, it helps if the doctor is quick-witted. But, of course, not all doctors have this gift. The next best thing is to be prepared for the sort of question which may be asked. Here, experience helps.

Every doctor needs to be prepared to answer the question: *"Is it serious?"* In my experience, this comes more often from a relative than from the patient. The doctor must always err on the side of encouragement. He must never extinguish hope. My practice in dealing with the relative of a patient with a heart attack or heart failure or a stroke of moderate severity, in which I did not expect trouble, was to say:

> *"I think he should do well; but of course the first few days are likely to be rather anxious until we can see that he is making progress."*

If the outcome was more doubtful, I would say:

> *"Of course, he is seriously ill; but I think he should pull round all right."*

If the situation looked desperate, I would say:

> *"Things are critical; but not hopeless."*

Lord Dawson used to say, in such circumstances, *"So far so good"*, often adding under his breath *"but not very far"*.

There are certain words, such as cancer and leukaemia, which have such an ominous ring to a layman that I never used them unless I could say truthfully: *"You haven't got cancer (or leukaemia) if that is what you are worried about."* If a patient with cancer asked me outright if he had it, I made it my practice to tell him the truth. But I always tried to soften the impact by adding something encouraging, for example *"Fortunately, it is one of the treatable kinds"* or *"Fortunately, it is not one of the most serious kinds"* or, if it is in an advanced state, *"We will not let you suffer"*. It is worth bearing in mind that many types of cancer have occasionally been reported to have entered a phase of spontaneous regression[5].

There is one sentence which a doctor should never pronounce, and that is: *"I can't do any more for you."* It extinguishes hope. Furthermore, it is never true. There is always something more to be tried, however unpromising it may seem. The doctor may, however, have to tell a patient with a chronic disability that he will have to live with it.

Sometimes the patient volunteers a remark which the doctor feels he needs to correct. A grateful patient may say: *"Thank you, doctor; I know I owe it all to you."* Of course, it is well meant, but it is not true, and I do not think we should let it pass. Usually, other health care professionals have been involved. But, on a Christian view, the patient owes his healing to God's blessing of whatever means were used, and I think the doctor should say so. One of the doctors' besetting temptations is pride, and we should readily admit our limitations.

Never criticise the general practitioner

Not infrequently, the patient invites the specialist to criticise other doctors: *"Don't you think my doctor ought to have spotted that?"* or *"Surely my doctor ought to have sent me to see you sooner?"* Sometimes the specialist is inclined to agree with the patient but it is almost never right to say so. One never knows the precise reason for the other doctor's mistake. He may have had to examine the patient in a poor light or in a noisy environment or in a sagging bed at home. What is so obvious now may not have been obvious earlier. Whatever the reason, we all make mistakes and we should treat others as we would wish to be treated ourselves. I am speaking of a colleague's isolated mistake. I do not consider it right to cover up for a doctor who is chronically incompetent or lazy.

Factors militating against good communication

One of the reasons why doctors are bad at communication is that, because their work is so demanding, they find it difficult to spare the time for effective communication. There is no denying that effective communication involves time and trouble, but it is time well spent. Doctors often fear that garrulous patients will waste their time. They can do, but the remedy is for the doctor to remain in control, and step in to put an end to any attempt to take advantage of his openness, pleasantly but firmly. The best guide in this, as in all aspects of patient management, is to say to oneself: *"How would I act if the patient was a respected member of my own family — my mother or father, wife or husband?"*

Another equally powerful reason why doctors tend to minimise conversation with patients is that communication makes the doctor vulnerable. There are many situations in which we have to admit that we do not know the precise diagnosis and, even more frequently, the prognosis. The more freely we communicate, the more often we shall be proved wrong! I have not forgotten an occasion when I had under my care a nursing officer with anaemia, caused by a slow haemorrhage from a duodenal ulcer. After several days, her condition appeared, at last, to have stabilised. Her relative was anxious, and I thought I ought to give her some reassurance. I did so, but that very evening the patient suffered a massive haemorrhage. Such experiences tend to discourage communication, but they should not do so. The lesson is to be guarded in one's reassurance in such circumstances.

Communication, concern and kindness cover a multitude of sins. Thus, even from the lowest consideration of avoiding trouble, it is essential that doctors strive to improve their communication skills.

Practical advice

A hospital chaplain with whom I had a long and fruitful association set out some good practical advice for doctors on this subject. His close contact with patients had impressed on him the inhibitory effect of the 'team' accompanying a consultant. He noted that too often the ward round left behind bewildered patients, bursting with unanswered questions. He insisted that the patient wants to speak to his doctor on a one-to-one basis. Patients do not, and will not, ask questions of a group of doctors, partly because they want privacy and partly because they are afraid of asking something obvious and stupid. Even intelligent and well-informed patients are somewhat in the situation of the African woman I met on a visit to her village. She asked me, through an interpreter, how we, in Britain, made use of dogs, and specifically of guide dogs. She could not understand how a dog could lead a blind person. *"Does the person catch hold of its tail?"* she asked. She had never seen a harness and lead.

I cannot do better than quote the advice of a surgical friend of mine on the subject of talking to patients. He recommended the following[6]:

◆ Look the patient in the eye.
◆ Get alongside the patient when you talk. Never attempt to converse from the foot of the bed.
◆ Speak slowly.
◆ Be human.
◆ Curb impatience.
◆ Beware of clichés like *"Don't worry"*, *"Take it easy"*, and *"You'll be all right"*.
◆ Always keep a step ahead. Anticipate your patient's next probable anxiety.
◆ Keep to the truth.
◆ Beware of arrogance.

Aids to communication

Because of the importance of the doctor's advice, and the difficulty most patients have in retaining it, it has been suggested that the essence of his instructions should be available to the patient in written form. This can be done in the case of common problems. Indeed, many specialist patients' associations provide helpful explanatory leaflets. On the other hand, no prepared hand-out can cater fully for the individual needs of patients. In my own practice, 48 hours before discharging a patient after a heart attack, I would give him a booklet about his condition, and offer to answer any questions after he had read it. This seemed to work well.

One way round the difficulty that patients have in recalling the specialist's advice is for them to see the letter to the referring doctor, or receive a copy of it, simplified and edited if necessary. Another suggestion, of which I have no experience, is for the doctor to give the patient an audio-recording of what he has told him. The patient can then play it back to himself (and his family) at leisure in his home. Some immigrant patients cannot read English, and a few cannot even read their native language. For such patients, audio-tapes may be invaluable.

Some warnings

Doctors must remember that patients easily misunderstand casual remarks. A friend of my wife's was in hospital for surgery, and a midwife with uterine bleeding lay in the next bed. The surgeon visited the midwife after her operation and said:

> "*We did the hysterectomy as planned, and took out your ovaries as well. You won't need them. They were rotten.*"

The patient brooded over the word 'rotten', unable to ask what the surgeon meant. She was afraid, not simply of looking stupid, but of what she might hear.

A doctor must be careful that remarks which are not intended for the patient cannot be overheard by the patient and misinterpreted, as happens all too easily. A consultant had just examined a patient who had been operated on by his assistant. He said nothing to the patient, but outside the door of her room he proceeded to make critical comments about her postoperative care, which the patient overheard. She was naturally very upset. Sometimes a doctor teaching at the bedside will make an amusing comment to liven up the student teaching. The danger is that, all too easily, the patient may conclude that the laughter is at his expense.

It is important to recognise that hearing is just about the last of the senses to be lost, both under anaesthesia and before death. Because an obstetrician overlooked this fact he found himself being sued by a woman he had delivered by forceps under general anaesthesia. She claimed that she had been inadequately anaesthetised, and she supported her claim by saying that as the obstetrician delivered her baby, she heard him exclaim: *"Damn it. After all the trouble, the baby is as ugly as its mother!"*

A remarkable example was reported in the *Church Times* a few years ago. A vicar was called to the bedside of an elderly widow, who was unconscious and had been pronounced close to death by the doctor. The vicar became convinced that she would not die. He said as much over her inert body and prayed for healing. She later recovered and related every word of the bedside conversation[7]. So we need to be careful what we say in the presence of the seemingly unconscious.

References

1. Holmes OW (1891) *Medical Essays*. Samson Low, London: 389

2. Ley P (1983) Patients' understanding and recall in clinical communication failure. In: Pendleton D, Hasler J, eds. *Doctor/Patient Communication*. Academic Press, London: 94

3. Maheswaran CM (1994) Happiness regained (Personal view). *Br*

Med J **308**: 925

4. Levinson W (1994) Physician/patient communication: a key to malpractice prevention (editorial). *JAMA* **272**: 1619–20

5. Boyd W (1966) *The Spontaneous Regression of Cancer*. Charles C. Thomas, Springfield, Illinois

6. Scorer CG (1980) Talking with patients. In: Vale A, ed. *Medicine and the Christian Mind, 2nd edn*. Christian Medical Fellowship, London: 59–63

7. Minerva (1991) *Br Med J* **302**: 1162

Chapter 7
THE ART OF GOOD PRESCRIBING

◆ Iatrogenic disease
◆ Ensuring compliance
◆ Warning about side-effects
◆ Choice of remedy
◆ Use of placebos
◆ Learning from international differences in prescribing

In the matter of prescribing, the specialist must recognise that he is at a disadvantage by comparison with the general practitioner on two counts. First, he is not so familiar with the patient's history of drug reactions. Secondly, he does not have the same opportunity to monitor the patient's response to the treatment he advises, and to adjust the dose or replace the drug of first choice by another.

There are four aims that a prescriber should try to achieve, both on first prescribing a drug and on subsequently monitoring it. They are: to maximise effectiveness, minimise risks, minimise costs and respect the patient's choices[1].

Iatrogenic disease

Doctors have a reputation for overstating the benefits and understating the risks of the drugs they prescribe. There was a time when a physician could safely prescribe a more or less innocuous preparation for any complaint. That day has passed. Nevertheless, many patients still want a prescription and often specify the class of drug they want, for example. an antibiotic, a hypnotic or a non-steroidal anti-inflammatory drug. The doctor may be tempted to prescribe something in order to satisfy the patient and shorten the consultation, without stopping to consider whether it is rational or indeed safe.

It cannot be denied that there has been a lot of over-prescribing in the past, and it is likely that it continues. This faulty practice has led to a considerable amount of iatrogenic disease. Such disease is often mild, but is frequently unpleasant and occasionally fatal. This is particularly so in the case of misguided or inadequately controlled use of corticosteroids and anticoagulants. It was recently calculated that as many as 240 000 patients were admitted to hospital annually with diseases resulting wholly or largely from adverse reactions to drugs[2]. Since drug reactions are often unrecognised, and rarely reported, the true figures may be as much as ten times higher than those quoted.

It is important to ascertain what medicines a patient is already taking before prescribing a new drug, and always to check for possible drug interaction — by an appropriately programmed computer, if this is available. It is also important always to ask about allergies and never to ignore them, although the patient's ideas cannot invariably be accepted at face value.

Ensuring compliance

Although many patients still demand drugs, an increasing number go to the other extreme and refuse them. Sometimes it is difficult to persuade a patient to take an essential remedy. Unless this can be done, the patient may reluctantly accept the prescription, and even obtain the drug (especially if it is free), but then leave it untouched.

As many as 40% of patients fail to follow advice regarding medication. Up to 20% do not even collect their prescriptions. Others do so, but then fail to take the drug[3,4]. One consequence of this is seen in the bathroom cupboards of thousands of homes, where bottles of tablets lie discarded; this represents a major waste of money and a potential source of danger to children and to the depressed. Non-compliance may be unintentional, due to forgetfulness or misunderstanding, but often it is intentional.

Compliance is powerfully influenced by the patient's level of satisfaction with the consultation[5].

Many patients start a course of treatment but give it up because of side-effects or because they are feeling better or they feel that the drug is doing them no good. This latter reason is particularly true of those with depressive illness. Patients who have no symptoms find it difficult to understand why they should continue with a treatment which makes them feel no better, and may even make them feel worse — as in the case of antihypertensive therapy. Careful explanation is needed to ensure compliance.

Warning patients against side-effects

In addition to explaining the purpose of the treatment prescribed, it is essential to warn the patient against both common and important side-effects, particularly the possibility of drowsiness affecting driving and working with machines. It is, however, often difficult to know how far to go without making matters worse by suggestion. Few patients need to know all the possible side-effects, and few have sufficient understanding of the balance between benefit and risk to evaluate the doctor's recommendation. An elderly lady with bronchitis complicated by a depressive illness asked her sister to read out the side-effects of the antidepressive drug which she had been prescribed. When she heard that one of the side-effects listed was breathlessness, she decided not to take the drug.

Ideally, every patient should receive written instructions giving the name of each drug prescribed, when to take it, and its intended effect. A high proportion of patients are uncertain on one or more of these points. How to present the possible side-effects in a balanced way needs careful thought. Ideally, the patient should be able to exercise faith in his physician.

Everyone reacts differently to drugs, so that the dosage must be tailored to the patient more carefully than has been the practice in the past. For example, the patient might be told to start with a certain dose, and halve it if it produces intolerable side-effects. Alternatively, he may be told to start with a small dose, and double it until it has the desired effect.

Sometimes, it is very difficult to know how to strike the right balance between relief of symptoms and the presence of side-effects. This is particularly so in treatment involving corticosteroids. A patient with rheumatoid arthritis[6] was able to lead a completely normal life, including sporting activities, whilst she was taking high doses of steroids. But her face became grossly cushingoid to the extent that she could not bear to look at herself in the mirror. A slight graze turned into a large laceration which refused to heal. Her weight fluctuated by four or five pounds per day, she felt moody, and her blood pressure rose. She decided the price was too high and asked to come off steroids. She lost her mobility, and did not know how she would manage if the disease progressed, but she felt she was back in control of her body and mind, and more at peace with herself.

Particular care is necessary in prescribing at both ends of life. The administration of an inappropriately large dose to a child may be fatal and has been the ruin of some promising careers. Prescribing for the elderly is equally hazardous, since many are especially sensitive to both the intended and the unintended effects of drugs. Moreover, the compliance of the elderly is impaired by poor memory, poor vision and poor hearing.

Compliance decreases dramatically with the number of tablets prescribed. Prescribing is frequently too complex, with some medicines to be taken 8-hourly, some 6-hourly, and others less frequently. A mathematician would find it difficult to obey the instructions precisely. For those who are old and confused, even approximate compliance is impossible. There are several ways round this situation. One is to compromise, and modify the timing of the different drugs so that the patient has to remember to take his drugs only twice, or at the most three times, in the day. Another is to provide the patient with a pill box (Dosette) that has compartments labelled clearly to show the time of day for each tablet or capsule. A third method is to make use of combined tablets. This device is beloved by drug companies and general practitioners but has, in the past, been abhorred by hospital consultants because of the difficulty of adjusting drug doses individually, and because of suboptimal timing of ingestion.

Choice of remedy

It goes without saying that the doctor should take the cost of the remedy into account. This is so whether the payment comes directly from the patient or from some other source. Although many doctors reject guidelines in prescribing as 'cook-book medicine', there is much to be said for them, provided that they are simply guidelines and not mandatory decrees. It is certainly valuable to have up-to-date information regarding relative costs of commonly used remedies such as diuretics, antihypertensives, antidepressives and non-steroidal anti- inflammatory drugs.

The doctor must have confidence in the drug he prescribes. In the past, there has been a problem over the quality of some products, and some physicians are still concerned about the bioequivalence of drugs which purport to have identical effects[7]. Generic prescribing undoubtedly saves expense, and should be encouraged in principle[8]. However, it carries the risk that patients on maintenance therapy may be confused by being given a tablet of unfamiliar appearance when their prescription is repeated.

When should new and relatively untried remedies be used? Obviously, when older and established remedies have failed. But restraint is needed. Sir Robert Hutchison wrote:

> *"It is usually wise to be a little behind the fashion in matters of treatment."*[9]

Such a practice minimises the danger of getting caught out by a new drug with serious side-effects which are slow to come to light. Alexander Pope's advice is applicable to the art of prescribing:

> *"Be not the first by whom the new is tried;*
> *Nor yet the last to lay the old aside."*

There are some patients who despise inexpensive remedies and are only satisfied by expensive ones. There are others who claim to react badly to every remedy that is tried. Such patients present a great problem. In the case of private patients, I have sometimes succeeded by replacing a drug which the patient has rejected, by an equivalent drug bearing an unfamiliar name, for example digoxin by lanatoside C or Cedilanid.

The use of placebos

A placebo has been defined as any treatment deliberately used for non-specific psychological or psychophysiological effect[10]. It has been claimed that the use of a placebo involves deception because the patient thinks he is being given something which will alleviate his symptoms when, in fact, he is being given a preparation which, if not strictly 'inactive', is nevertheless without specific activity for the condition being treated.

In a sense every doctor uses a placebo continuously simply by virtue of his position of authority in our culture. The most powerful placebo force in medical practice is the physician himself — what Balint[11] called 'the doctor drug'. The doctor's confident manner in recommending whatever treatment he advocates has therapeutic value. When a new drug comes on the scene, the doctor's enthusiasm may enhance its effect. Hence, Osler's advice to *"treat as many patients as possible with a new drug while it still has the power to heal."*

Until recently, there were few drugs which were really effective, and much of therapeutics consisted in the wise use of placebos, although most of the doctors who prescribed them believed that they were active preparations and consequently no ethical problem arose.

As to whether the deliberate prescription of a placebo is ethical, I am inclined to agree with the conclusions reached by the medical study group of the Christian Medical Fellowship; namely that if a placebo is used as a means of fobbing off a patient, it is wrong, but if it is used as a means of bringing relief without harming the patient, then it is legitimate. The essential considerations are, first that the treatment which is prescribed should help the patient, not only in the short-term but also in the long-term and, secondly, that the doctor should not deceive himself[12].

Many orthodox doctors believe that most of the benefit which is claimed to result from the use of homeopathy and other forms of alternative medicine is a placebo effect. Even if this is the case, it should not necessarily be used as an argument for the wholesale rejection of alternative therapies. If the treatment actually does the patient good in the long term, it cannot readily be dismissed, even if the theory behind its use is implausible. Certainly, an alternative practitioner who sincerely believes in the efficacy of his form of treatment cannot be charged with duplicity; and his confidence, even if it is misplaced, undoubtedly plays some part in its success.

It has been pointed out that for many patients, the potency of a remedy is enhanced by some sign. It may be a strong taste, or a harmless side-effect such as a dry mouth or coloured urine. A distinctive appearance, such as a spangled capsule or a tablet of unusual shape, seems to be more effective than an ordinary-looking preparation.

International differences in prescribing

There is a wide variation in prescribing habits from one country to another[13], which is perpetuated by the teaching that medical students receive in the course of their training. In general, British general practitioners prescribe far fewer drugs than do most of their European counterparts[14]. Thus, while French patients receive 38 items on prescription per annum, British patients receive less than eight. Furthermore, British doctors are more likely to offer older and less expensive medication, appearing to be more cautious and money conscious. The French government has recently published guidelines for prescribing, aimed at ensuring that doctors do not systematically over-prescribe. They can now be fined for doing so[15].

These international differences are worthy of closer study than they have yet received, because there are lessons to be learned and, possibly, some savings to be made. They undoubtedly indicate a degree of uncertainty regarding the best treatment for some conditions. The French are, to our view, obsessed with their livers and consume many medicines directed at the gastrointestinal tract. They also use a lot of cerebral vasodilators and tonics. So far as conventional remedies are concerned, it is noteworthy that their doses are often only half those used in Britain, in accordance with their policy of employing 'les medicines douces'. The Germans are obsessed with 'cardiac insufficiency' and prescribe six times the amount of cardiac drugs compared with Britain and France. They also diagnose low blood pressure far more often than we do, and have scores of drugs for its treatment.

The form of preparation which 'pleases' a patient varies from country to country. In some countries, tablets and medicines are despised and the patient only has faith in injections and suppositories.

References

1. Barbes N (1995) What constitutes good prescribing? *Br Med J* 310: 923–5

2. Medawar C (1992) *Power and Dependence: Social Audit on the Safety of Medicines*. Social Audit Ltd, London: 3

3. Aronson JK, Hardman M (1992) Patient compliance. *Br Med J* 305: 1009–10

4. Beardon PHG, McGilchrist MM, McKendrick AD, McDevitt DG, MacDonald TM (1993) Primary non-compliance with prescribed medication in primary care. *Br Med J* 307: 846–8

5. Ley P (1983) Patients' understanding and recall in clinical communication failure. In: Pendleton D and Hasler J, eds. *Doctor/Patient Communication*. Academic Press, London: 102

6. Personal View (1994) The story of an illness. *Br Med J* 309: 1448

7. Pearson M *et al* (1994) Generic inhalers for asthma (letter). *Br Med J* 309: 1440

8. Gilley J (1994) Towards rational prescribing. *Br Med J* 308: 731–2

9. Hutchison R (1940) *Index of Treatment*. Wright, Bristol: 2

10. Oh VMS (1994) The placebo effect: can we use it better? *Br Med J* **309**: 69–70

11. Balint M (1964) *The Doctor, His Patient and the Illness*. Pitman, London

12. Fergusson A (1988). Alternative medicine — a review. *J Christian Med Fellowship* **34**: 26–9

13. Payer L (1988) *Medicine and Culture: Varieties of Treatment in the US, England, West Germany and France*. Henry Holt and Co, New York

14. Griffin JP, Griffin TD (1993) The economic implications of therapeutic conservatism. *J R Coll Physicians Lond* **27**: 121–6

15. Dorozynski A (1994) French Government issues guidelines on prescriptions. *Br Med J* **308**: 1002

Chapter 8
CASE NOTES AND LETTERS

◆ Importance of an accurate contemporaneous record
◆ Practical tips on note taking
◆ Confidentiality
◆ What to include in the letter to the referring doctor
◆ What to avoid
◆ Eliminating delays in communication

Case notes

Importance

An accurate record of every consultation is essential. In the first place, it forms the basis of the letter to the referring doctor. Secondly, it is essential to any future personal involvement with the patient. Even the best of memories is fallible for dates and details, such as blood pressure readings, and it is only too easy to confuse one patient with another. A detailed record, made at the time, is also essential in view of the team work involved in modern medical practice. It is very likely that another doctor will see the patient on a subsequent occasion and will need to know the background history, what the patient complained of, what was found on examination and the results of any investigations. Equally, an accurate record is essential if the notes are to be used for research purposes.

Above all, an accurate record, written at the time of examination, is crucial in the event of the patient making a complaint about his management. The Medical Defence Union[1] recommends that the doctor should document details, such as the patient's denial of allergies or other contraindications to therapy, and also record any warnings of side-effects given to the patient. If another doctor is consulted, his name should be recorded. There is a strong temptation for doctors to make inadequate notes on domiciliary visits.

Practical suggestions

My practice was to jot down notes while the patient was speaking, using my own abbreviations, and to supplement these with further notes, either written or dictated into an electronic recorder, while the patient was undressing for examination. I wrote up the definitive record on the history and examination at the earliest opportunity and, when possible, had it typed.

In future, abbreviations may be standardised. The National Health Service Centre for Coding and Classification is working on a 'Clinical Terms Project' to create a set of acceptable abbreviations for recording clinical data, with a view to facilitating the computerisation of medical records[2].

It is highly desirable, if not essential, for the examination room to be separate from the consulting room. This allows the doctor to make further notes without being interrupted by the patient calling out additional points of history or informing the doctor that he is ready to be examined. It also gives the doctor the opportunity to consult some source of information, e.g. by computer, or to speak briefly with a colleague or another patient without being overheard.

Confidentiality

Care is necessary to avoid including in the records observations which might cause unnecessary anxiety or give offence if the patient demanded to see them. This creates a problem, because doctors need somewhere to record candid, uninhibited impressions, comments, speculations and reminders[3]. Moreover, there are, arguably, some matters which are so personal and upsetting for the patient that they should not be shared with anyone else, or even recorded in the notes[4]. It is difficult to see how the doctor can do this without retaining a confidential *aide-mémoire*.

It is important to do everything possible to preserve the confidentiality of the patient's case notes. In one group general practice, it was calculated that 40 people other than doctors had access to patients' records — all with good reason[5]. Similar, if somewhat less extensive, access may well be possible at the present time in many hospitals. As Horner has pointed out, an individual's information could, potentially, be shared with the largest workforce in Europe[6]. It is highly unlikely that a patient realises this when he confides in his doctor.

Potential for clinical research

If outpatient consultations are to be used as a basis for clinical research, the first step is to identify a problem which crops up frequently. The next is to design a proforma for such cases, try it out and amend it so that there are no gaps in the data base. The completed proforma should, of course, be filed separately from the routine clinical notes. I also kept a separate file for 'diagnostic puzzles', retaining a copy of the case summary and hospital record number for later review.

In the future, the recording of notes is likely to be facilitated and accelerated by refinements in speech-recognition computer systems.

Letter to the referring doctor

Communication between doctors must be clear, accurate, courteous and prompt. The letter referring the patient to the specialist should indicate the problem which occasions the consultation, and mention relevant points which the specialist may not discover by his questioning of the patient. It should include current medication, past drug intolerance, known allergies, any abnormal findings on investigation and any relevant sociopsychological matters. Frequently, as Hodge *et al*[7] found, *"the specific indication for referral is either unstated, distorted or lost in transmission"*. This results in a consultation which is less than satisfactory both for the patient and for the general practitioner.

The letter from the specialist to the referring doctor should report the positive findings and any significant negative findings. It should indicate the diagnosis or, failing that, the differential diagnosis, state any further investigations which may be needed, and what arrangements are being made for this and for follow-up. The letter should give advice about treatment, report what the patient was told, and indicate any surprising reaction to this information. If the referring doctor asked a specific question, this should of course be answered. If the consultant does not know the answer, he should not be ashamed to admit it. He should also give an indication as to when he would expect the patient to be able to return to work, while recognising that the general practitioner knows more about the patient's circumstances than does the specialist. He should also make it clear under what circumstances the patient should be referred back to him.

There is a difference of opinion as to whether the consultant's letter should set out the history in full. Some think it should do so for the benefit of other doctors who may be called upon to review the patient at a later date[8]. Personally, I did not do this, on the grounds that the referring doctor should know the history better than the specialist and that, in any case, the history was recorded in full in the case notes. This meant that the letter could be kept brief.

The specialist's letter should avoid the danger of claiming too much credit for an apparently successful outcome. Sir James Howie told the story of one of the consultants for whom he worked as a house physician. He had admitted to hospital a patient from 40 miles out in the country with atrial fibrillation, who was restored to sinus rhythm by the use of quinidine. The house physician wrote the discharge letter, setting out the bare facts. The consultant, however, was not satisfied and replaced it by his own letter. It went along the following lines:

> *"Dear Dr ... We treated your patient, who had atrial*
> *fibrillation, with quinidine, and he made an excellent*
> *recovery. Indeed, I would regard him as one of my*

most successful cases. "

The patient duly took this letter in his pocket and set off for home. Unfortunately he collapsed and died before he had got very far. The police found the letter in his pocket, went to see the consultant, saying something to the effect:

> *"Doctor; This patient just got as far as the railway station before he died. How far do your less successful cases get?"*

Conveying bad news

In Britain, the patient is entitled to see all his records and the relevant correspondence, so that the consultant may feel some reservation as to what he writes concerning a patient whose prognosis is poor. In the past, he was able to write honestly, and leave it to the family doctor's discretion how to answer the patient's questions. This is still, in my view, the ideal arrangement. However much the consultant may have told the patient, the general practitioner is likely to be asked to elaborate and to discuss points which had not occurred to the patient at the time of his consultation with the specialist. This puts the onus on the general practitioner to handle any request by the patient to see the letter. Fortunately, such a request is uncommon.

What to avoid

Care must be taken to avoid offensive remarks. Even such an opening statement as *"I saw your charming patient at my clinic this afternoon"* (which used to introduce many a specialist's letter in the past, especially in relation to a private patient!) has been criticised as being unduly patronising. Ideally, letters should be interesting and a pleasure to read, although attempts at humour are fraught with danger.

The importance of a prompt reply

It is important to reply to the referring doctor without delay. It is most unsatisfactory if, as still happens all too often, the patient returns to the general practitioner before the specialist's report has been received. The consultant should dictate (or type) his letter immediately after seeing the patient, if at all possible. If the results of crucial investigations are expected within 48 hours, dictation might be delayed to take account of them, or the results may be added as a postscript. If results cannot be expected for several days, an interim letter should be sent, or a provisional report communicated by telephone to the general practitioner or his secretary. Speed in getting a letter to the referring doctor is helped by brevity. Many specialists' letters are verbose.

Delay between typing and signing should be cut to a minimum. If the consultant is due to go on holiday or to a conference, an experienced and reliable secretary can be asked to initial the letter and indicate that it was dictated but not checked by the specialist. If the letter includes a critical dose of a powerful drug, it should be scrutinised by a competent medical assistant.

Postal delays can be eliminated by electronic transmission between hospital and health centre computers, or by faxing — provided that the information is not of a sensitive nature. It is often appropriate, when discharging a patient from hospital, to hand him a copy of the brief interim discharge letter, giving the diagnosis and treatment, which he can take to his doctor at his next attendance. Another copy should be sent by post, and a further one retained in the hospital notes. Occasionally, the specialist may give the patient a handwritten letter to take back to his general practitioner. This should be done on self-copying paper so that there is a record for the notes.

There is currently a move towards the greater use of structured letters. There is some evidence that general practitioners prefer these to conventional letters[9]. Structured letters have the advantage that they oblige the writer to state concisely what he thinks the patient's problems are and how they should be managed. They also enable the reader to see at a glance what the writer's views are.

Moreover, they are shorter and enable general practitioners to transfer information more easily to computerised patient records.

References

1. Guly HF (1993) Medico-legal problems in accident and emergency departments. *J Med Defence Union* 9: 36–9

2. Clarke JA (1994) A new era in clinical information? Read codes and the terms projects. *Proc R Coll Physicians Edinb* 24: 360–3

3. Short D (1986) Some consequences of granting patients access to consultants' records. *Lancet* i: 1316–18

4. Elliott-Binns C (1978) *Medicine — the Forgotten Art*. Pitman Medical, 107

5. Markus A, Lockwood M (1991) Is it permissible to edit medical records? *Br Med J* 303: 349–51

6. Horner S (1994) Confidentiality. *Nucleus* **April**: 5

7. Hodge JAH, Jacob A, Ford MJ, Munro JF (1992) Medical clinic referral letters. Do they say what they mean? Do they mean what they say? *Scott Med J* 37: 179–180

8. Lipworth BJ, Allan J, Jackson CM, Dhillon PD, Winter JH, Clark RA (1993) An audit of hospital discharge letters in patients admitted with acute asthma. *Scott Med J* 38: 116–9

9. Rawal J, Barnett P, Lloyd BW (1993) Use of structured letters to improve communication between hospital doctors and general practitioners. *Brit Med J* 307: 1044

Chapter 9
WHEN LITTLE CAN BE DONE

◆ Chronic illness
◆ Incurable disease
◆ When to seek a second opinion
◆ Considering 'alternative' therapies
◆ When not to resuscitate
◆ Caring for the carer

This chapter faces problems that arise when the consultant encounters situations which he cannot influence decisively, such as chronic handicap, incurably progressive disease and patients in the terminal phase of life.

No-one likes to be reminded of failure. This is as true of doctors as of anyone else. Yet the doctor cannot always be successful. Often his treatment can only be palliative. Frequently, even this limited goal may not be attainable, such as when the disease proves to be more extensive than he realised, when complications such as infection, stroke or pulmonary embolism develop, or when the side-effects of drugs make it so.

Chronic illness

It is essential for the consultant to realise that his work has a 'caring' as well as a 'curing' dimension. It may not be the task of the physician or surgeon to provide the caring, but it is certainly his responsibility to arrange for it. *"Guerir quelquefois, soulager souvent, consoler toujours"* sums up the doctor's calling.

The patient must be helped to accept chronic illness. The following advice (attributed to Tuker) is applicable to a wide range of unremitting and limiting diseases:

"Whoever has the care of a sorely stricken arthritic must encourage him to fulfil himself intellectually and

*spiritually, and to achieve — no matter what, but to
achieve, so that he may nightly lay himself down on his
bed of pain looking forward happily to the morrow's
task, mind centred upon it, no matter what it is;
sticking in stamps, research into anything you like,
dabbling with pastel or water colours, writing chatty
letters to friends. Anything at all, but let it be for him
the most pressing thing of the day, and let him believe
that you think it is. Help him and let him live, live
fully."*

Incurable disease

When it has become clear that cure, and even significant relief, can
no longer be hoped for, there is a tendency for the doctor's interest
in the patient to wane. This can be seen on the ward round. The
patient who was once the focus of constant interest and a star
subject for student teaching has become a 'heart-sink' patient. The
consultant is only too happy if this patient is behind screens when
he is doing his round. The patient, deserted by the consultant, and
left in the hands of inexperienced doctors, is deprived of adequate
care and analgesia. The specialist has a responsibility to help the
patient to the very end of the road.

In dealing with patients suffering from incurable disease,
especially cancer, there is a tendency to adopt an automatic
reassuring attitude to their symptoms. When a patient who has had
a laparotomy or palliative surgery complains of a pain, it is easy to
dismiss it with: *"Well, it is only to be expected after a big operation."*
Often, the patient's complaint expresses a fear or anxiety about
something to which, if the doctor approached it more
sympathetically, he could give a more convincing reassurance. It is
better to ask the patient what the pain feels like, uncover the
underlying anxiety, and then reassure. Often, patients' fears are
based on a simple misunderstanding. Once this is dealt with,
reassurance is much more effective.

A positive attitude is to be encouraged. The patient should be
urged to take every day as it comes, in the knowledge that the

course of cancer is uncertain and fluctuating, and that even advanced cancer has occasionally been reported as remitting[1].

Alternative therapies

Many patients refuse to accept a diagnosis of incurable disease and are determined to 'fight' it. They may ask their doctor's advice about consulting an alternative therapist. The idea should not be rejected out of hand. Complementary therapies have been found to give symptomatic help to patients going through the trauma of chemotherapy and radiotherapy[2]. On the other hand, patients should be warned against wasting their money on the latest 'cancer cure'. They can be assured that whenever a treatment of proven value is found, the medical profession will recognise and adopt it.

Seeking a second opinion

When should the specialist suggest referring the patient for a second opinion? The first point to make is that it is far better for the doctor to offer it than to wait until the patient demands it. A survey in *Which? Way to Health*[3] revealed that the commonest reasons for a patient requesting a second opinion were that current treatment did not seem to be working, a need for reassurance, lack of confidence in the doctor's expertise, and lack of information about their condition.

A specialist is, by definition, not an expert in all diseases. Therefore, if the patient's main need is for the correct diagnosis and management of a disease in which the consultant is inexpert, and an appropriate specialist is available, it stands to reason that the patient would do better to be transferred under his care. In my experience, there is a strong temptation to hang on to patients with interesting diseases, in order to enlarge one's experience or to have an unusual patient for teaching or, in the case of private practice, for financial reasons. Nevertheless, the key consideration must be the patient's best interests. Sometimes, all that is necessary is to call in a colleague for consultation, while retaining overall control.

My practice was to propose a second opinion quite freely. I

can only remember one patient having to request such a course, although there have certainly been others for whom I had not made a correct diagnosis or whom I had not succeeded in satisfying, and who went elsewhere. It is important not to allow oneself to be offended by such things. The patient's welfare is more important that the consultant's self-esteem. When a doctor does request a second opinion, he should make clear to his colleague whether it is primarily for advice or for action.

When not to resuscitate

Sometimes the patient asks the doctor to end his life. Such a request should be received seriously and sympathetically. If it arises from an intractable symptom such as pain or nausea, the doctor should re-double his efforts to relieve it, even if in so doing he hastens his patient's demise. Every consultant, whatever his specialty, has a duty to keep up to date with the latest advances in symptom relief. Those practising in Great Britain are fortunate in that, thanks to the hospice movement, there is increasingly widespread provision for the relief of chronic pain, for terminal care, and also for advice. So-called 'mercy killing', with all its superficial attraction, has been repeatedly rejected by most civilised countries, in my opinion rightly, in view of all the problems which would arise if it were to be legalised[4]. In general, Christians, like Jews and Moslems, respect the divine prohibition against the taking of human life (Genesis 9;5,6).

On the other hand, it is equally important to avoid futile action which only serves to prolong artificially a miserable existence. If a patient with advanced and incurable cancer suffers a cardiac arrest, the event should, in the absence of instructions to the contrary, be regarded as a merciful release. Much of the pressure for 'mercy killing' and much of the enthusiasm for the 'living will' arise from the perception that doctors all too often resuscitate patients unwisely, thereby prolonging a life of misery. The patient's current informed wishes should be ascertained and followed as far as possible, and all decisions should be taken in collaboration with the nursing staff and the patients' relatives.

When patients are incompetent, doctors must make choices about resuscitation in their best interests.

The ultimate decision to withdraw or withhold treatment lies with the medical and nursing staff caring for the patient. In the past, it has been considered essential to seek the advice of the next of kin. It is now recognised that, although they should be consulted, their wishes should not invariably be followed, for two reasons. In the first place, their decision may be the opposite of that which the patient would make. Secondly, the burden of making life or death decisions should not be placed on the shoulders of someone who is already under great stress[5]. Doyal and Wilsher[6] have recently proposed formal guidelines for withholding cardiopulmonary resuscitation.

Often, symptoms are intensified by social factors. The patient feels that he is a burden, or believes that he is rejected by his family. In such a situation, an attempt must be made to restore a sense of worth and dignity. This is where the hospice movement has been so successful. Investigation should not be pursued if the objective is purely academic. Curative treatment should not be continued if it is not contributing to relief of the patient's symptoms. Too often one comes across patients who are compelled to take a multiplicity of tablets in the last weeks of their life, long after their ineffectiveness has become obvious.

Tournier[7] emphasised the importance of giving the patient plenty of time to talk over his problems with a good listener. Sometimes he found himself in a position in which he could best help the patient by drawing on his own experience, both of frustration and rebellion in the face of restrictions, and also, speaking as a Christian, of the strength he had found in faith and prayer. Jews and Christians share a common heritage in the immortal Psalms of David with their confident affirmations, such as: *"The Lord is my Shepherd, I shall not want"* (Psalm 23) and *"God is our refuge and strength, an ever present help in trouble"* (Psalm 46).

The consultant's responsibility for the carer

The doctor has a responsibility for the chronically ill patient's relatives and friends. Chalmers[8] has said:

> "Not infrequently I find that one of the most helpful things I can do for the carer is to accept full responsibility for the decision to pass the burden of care to someone else saying, in essence: 'You are not "putting her away". I am telling you that she must come into hospital, and that is my decision, not yours.'"

He sometimes uses the shortage of hospital beds to reinforce his advice: "I wouldn't take her if it wasn't essential."

References

1.   Boyd W (1966) *The Spontaneous Regression of Cancer*. Charles C
        Thomas, Springfield, Illinois

2.   Burch C (1993) Alternatives on the N.H.S. *Which? Way to
        Health*: 125–7

3.   Rigge M (1991) Second opinions. *Which? Way to health*: 32–5

4.   Keown J (1992) The law and practice of euthanasia in The
        Netherlands. *Ethics & Medicine* **8**: 34–8

5.   Finer S, Theaker N, Raper R, Fisher M (1994) Surrogates'
        decisions in resuscitation are of limited value (letter). *Br Med J*
        309: 953

6.   Doyal L, Wilsher D (1994) Withholding and withdrawing
        life-sustaining treatment from elderly people: towards formal
        guidelines. *Br Med J* **308**: 1689–92

7.   Tournier P (1954) *A Doctor's Casebook in the Light of the Bible*.
        SCM Press, London: 178–185

8.   Chalmers G (1991) Growing old: the challenge of ageing. *J
        Christian Med Fellowship* **37**: 15–19

Chapter 10
DIFFICULT PATIENTS

- ◆ Difficult doctors
- ◆ Difficulties in diagnosis
- ◆ The 'fat file' group
- ◆ Malingerers
- ◆ Münchausen's syndrome
- ◆ How to manage difficult patients

Every doctor has a cluster of patients he classes as 'difficult', patients whose name on an appointment list or whose face in the waiting room makes his heart sink or his blood pressure rise. This chapter represents an attempt to help the consultant to handle such patients more successfully.

Difficult doctors

Although there are undoubtedly difficult patients, it is important to recognise that there are difficult doctors too. Many doctors are 'allergic' to deaf patients, or those with poor comprehension and command of the English language, or who are garrulous and rambling in their history, or who are dirty and unkempt; to those who have sexually transmitted disease, or are habitual smokers, or who have taken part in industrial action to the detriment of the health service. Some consultants are uninterested if a patient's needs do not fall within the area of his narrow research interests. These failings need to be recognised and rectified before focusing on difficult patients.

Why some patients are difficult

Patients may be difficult for a variety of reasons. A patient may be labelled difficult because of the circumstances in which he was first seen. Both doctor and patient may be frustrated by the late arrival of the ambulance conveying the patient to the clinic, or because the patient attended at the wrong place, so missing his appointment and arriving at the end of the clinic. (It is important not to overlook the possibility that what appears to be bad manners may, in fact, be evidence of cerebral dysfunction.) Much annoyance to both parties is caused by notes or X-rays which have gone astray. If the doctor appears ruffled or loses his temper on the first occasion, it is apt to sour relations for the future.

Difficulties in diagnosis

A common reason for a patient being classed as difficult is that the diagnosis is obscure. The specialist likes to be able to fit every patient into a definite diagnostic category. Often this cannot be done, at least at the first consultation. The doctor then feels vulnerable. He is afraid that the patient will demand to know the diagnosis before the doctor has reached it, and he will have to admit his ignorance. Patients are so regaled by the media with the triumphs of medical science that few have any idea how difficult diagnosis may be. Even the most experienced doctors have to admit failure from time to time. This is hardly surprising, because sometimes the cause of an illness is not clear even at necropsy.

Periodic attacks, analogous to what car mechanics would call 'an intermittent fault', may cause great difficulty in diagnosis. Physical symptoms that lack an obvious organic basis are common in medical practice. Many complaints of abdominal pain, dyspepsia, headache, backache, joint pain, chest pain, palpitations and fatigue fall into this category. Such patients consume much medical time. They are subjected to many fruitless investigations, and the end result is frequently unsatisfactory.

If there is a suspicion of organic disease, clearly this must be fully investigated. For example, a patient with a strong family history of coronary disease may complain of recurrent chest pain, which is not typical of angina but is nevertheless consistent with it. The doctor is placed in a difficult position. If he investigates the symptom thoroughly he may leave the patient with the impression that there is something seriously wrong, whether or not he is subsequently reassured. But if he fails to take it seriously, the outcome might be fatal.

When a doctor can find no organic disease to account for a patient's symptoms, he is tempted to regard them as neurotic — all 'in the mind.' If he is mistaken, the patient is doubly the loser. Not only do his symptoms continue unrelieved, but he also feels deeply misunderstood. The doctor has added insult to injury. This is well illustrated by a report which appeared in the *British Medical Journal*[1] a few years ago, under the heading: 'One doctor believed me'. A woman had suffered from symptoms of incontinence, constant pain, and bouts of vomiting after a hysterectomy. Over a period of 13 years, she had seen several specialists, and all of them had come to the same conclusion, namely that there was nothing wrong with her and that the best form of treatment would be the administration of a tranquilliser. As time went on, the patient faced an increasing amount of scepticism and 'humouring', summed up in advice such as: " *should go home and try to lead a normal life if I were you*". In a last desperate bid, when the patient was already beyond despair, she sought the help of a young consultant. He organised a series of tests, many of which she had already been through; eventually he was able to make a diagnosis which dispelled the myth of her being a psychosomatic case. The patient was told that, at the time of her hysterectomy, her bladder had been injured. Within a short space of time, she had further surgery, after which she was able to lead a normal life.

This true story is typical of many similar situations in which the patient has organic symptoms which the doctor is unable to account for and regards as neurotic. Examples abound in my experience. I think of the doctor's wife who collapsed to the floor in a busy shop and had to be taken home in a taxi, remaining prostrate with vertigo for a day or two afterwards. I recall the 17-year-old girl who was brought home by her driving instructor because she was unable to judge distances. She was ataxic on the stairs leading to her bedroom and later became unable to walk. Both these patients had acute illnesses, which were organic but were regarded as 'functional' by the specialist who first saw them. Both recovered completely and remain well 20 years later, but they cannot easily forgive the specialist's dismissive diagnosis of neurosis. I think also of the middle-aged widow who complained of persistent pain behind her left ear at a time when her only daughter was preparing to emigrate. Her symptoms too were regarded as 'supratentorial' until shortly before her death from oesophageal cancer.

It is a serious mistake to conclude that every patient who gives a history which is unsupported by physical signs or positive investigation must be neurotic. A leading article in the *British Medical Journal*[2] with the title 'Medically unexplained physical symptoms' put it well when it said:

> *"Many patients do not have a psychiatric disorder, though psychological factors (such as erroneous beliefs and anxiety) may affect their interpretation of minor physiological sensations. A multi-causal aetiology is most likely, with physical and psychological factors interacting."*

If there is no clear evidence of psychological disorder, it is best for the doctor to admit that he does not, at present, know the cause of the symptom, and to arrange to see the patient again after an interval. He can explain that the situation may have become clearer by then, or that he may, in the interval, have come across a report of a patient with similar symptoms. If the condition is incapacitating or potentially serious and remains obscure after further investigation, he should consider admission for observation or offer to arrange a second opinion (see chapter 9).

Failure to respond to treatment tends to make a doctor regard a patient as difficult. The doctor feels a sense of failure and is inclined to suspect the patient of not having adhered to the regimen prescribed.

The 'fat file' group

A small minority of difficult patients fall into the category variously designated the 'fat file' or 'fat envelope' group, or 'heart-sink' patients. Every doctor who has been in practice for a few years can go to his file and pull out sets of notes which are ten times thicker than those of the average patient. One doctor in general practice identified 28 heart-sink patients on his list: 22 female and six male. Nineteen of the 28 had no evidence of any significant medical disease, and attended frequently with multiple vague symptoms for which they refused to accept reassurance. The remaining nine had a background of severe medical disease, but their symptoms were bizarre and unlike those of organic disease[3]. Many patients with unexplained chronic abdominal pain and post-accident neurosis fall into the heart-sink category.

Most of these patients have seen several hospital specialists and have had scores of laboratory tests and X-ray examinations. The difficulty in managing these patients is compounded by the fact that, inevitably, they cannot always see the same doctor. Indeed, the regular doctor is usually only too pleased when this happens! Each new doctor has to familiarise himself with the ever-growing set of notes, or else adopt some unsatisfactory temporising measure.

It is in this group of patients that reassurance presents the greatest difficulty, and this aggravates the feeling of an unsatisfactory consultation on both the doctor's and the patient's side. What encouragement, or indeed what information, can a doctor give to a patient with persistent symptoms pointing to physical disease and in whom the results of tests are repeatedly negative?

Chronic abdominal pain

This is a common cause of heart-sink. A review of a group of 20 such women, aged between 26 and 73 years, revealed that they had, between them, seen 142 different doctors. Fourteen patients had had a hysterectomy, three had had their gall bladder removed, and another three had had an appendicectomy. The group as a whole had also gone through 148 other investigations or surgical procedures. Forty per cent had also tried alternative medicine. All remained unrelieved[4].

Post-accident neurosis

Post-accident neurosis is a well-defined and intractable source of difficulty. A common example is the case of a man who sustains an injury to his back at work. He feels justified in claiming compensation. Settlement of such a claim involves a protracted legal process, with repeated medical examinations, and a continuing situation of conflict. The claimant emphasises his symptoms. The examiner finds either no abnormality, or an abnormality which is commonly symptomless. It has been noted over and over again that the symptom resists all attempts at treatment until the claim has been settled; thereafter it subsides quickly.

Subjects of medical misadventure

These form another group of difficult patients. Medical mishaps impose a strain on the doctor/patient relationship. If they are due to a mistake by the doctor, they also give rise to a feeling of guilt. It is now agreed that the doctor may, without admitting liability, show sympathy to the patient, explain the sequence of events, and do all he can to help him. If the mishap is clearly the fault of the doctor, he should not hesitate to apologise. It is now recognised that the vast majority of patients who seek redress through the courts do so, not to obtain damages but to obtain an explanation and an apology, in the hope that whatever the mistake was, it will not be so likely to happen again.

Malingerers

Some patients can only be described as malingerers, consciously and wilfully feigning physical illness for some personal advantage.

Compensation cases are an obvious example. Others, predominantly young women, fabricate illness in various ways[5]. For example, some pretend to have a fever by placing their thermometer next to a radiator or by exchanging their thermometer with that of another patient who is pyrexial. Others keep a wound open and then go to the doctor and complain that it will not heal. Others take a purgative and complain of diarrhoea, or take an anticoagulant and complain of bruising, or take an overdose of insulin and produce symptoms of hypoglycaemia. True malingering is uncommon, but the possibility must not be overlooked.

A 17-year-old girl of my acquaintance attended her general practitioner's surgery frequently with trivial complaints. So much so that the senior partner, an eminently reasonable doctor, regarded Ishbel (not her real name) as his main menace. He determined to avoid referring her to hospital. But one day the girl found a time when a locum was holding the fort. She complained to him of severe abdominal pain and was immediately referred to hospital as an emergency. No cause for the pain was found and she was promptly discharged. A few months later, Ishbel began work as a mother's help. One of the daughters of the family developed acute sinusitis, for which she was treated by her general practitioner. Ishbel took a great interest in the girl's symptoms and then changed to her doctor. She went to the new doctor complaining of the same symptoms as the daughter of the house, and duly returned home with a diagnosis of acute sinusitis and appropriate treatment. A month later, a frequent visitor to the house was suspected of appendicitis. Ishbel questioned her closely about her symptoms, and shortly afterwards attended the doctor's surgery complaining of similar abdominal pain. The doctor arranged a surgical outpatient appointment for her. Within a few days, however, the symptoms became worse and an emergency admission had to be arranged. Again, no cause for the pain was found. Eventually, a surgeon felt compelled to remove her appendix. But in spite of this, her symptoms continued to recur.

Münchausen's syndrome

The most extreme and notorious deceivers have been designated as having Münchausen's syndrome. These patients, nearly always men, gain admission to hospital for pretended symptoms, often pain in the abdomen, chest or head, for which they demand surgery. They undergo many investigations and submit to repeated operations. Once discharged, they make their way to another hospital, give a different name, proffer a fresh set of complaints and demand further surgery. Because they give a false name and conceal reference to their previous hospital admissions, the new staff have to go through all the investigations again. Amazingly, these patients willingly accept all the inconvenience and discomfort involved — even including craniotomy! One such patient was eventually documented as having had 207 hospital admissions over a period of 34 years. He discharged himself from hospital on 133 occasions, whenever he realised that the staff were beginning to detect his fraud. His earliest symptoms were of headache, neck stiffness and photophobia, for which he submitted to numerous lumbar punctures and many carotid arteriograms. Later he started complaining of acute abdominal pain, for which he underwent dozens of barium meals and barium enemas, and no less than four laparotomies. During his 207 admissions, he gave 22 different surnames and eight different first names[6].

Why do patients try to deceive doctors in this way? For some it is no doubt a game. They enjoy pitting their wit against the experts. Some intelligent patients with rare diseases actually know more about their disease than does the doctor, and they take pleasure in catching him out. For most it seems to be an attempt to evade responsibility. They prefer the comfort of being cared for by doctors and nurses (even though it may involve unpleasant investigation and treatment) to the difficulties and problems of everyday life. And, of course, they gain a certain kudos through being 'a difficult and interesting case'.

Cases of Münchausen's syndrome are not easy to spot, although a history of frequent travelling from place to place is a clue to the diagnosis. If a compulsory system of personal identification numbers (PINs)[7] were ever introduced, it would make it possible to trace a patient's previous history rapidly, and would thereby neutralise one of the main stratagems of these patients. The danger of misuse of such a system is obvious. However, it has been forecast that shortly everyone in Britain will be identified by a new NHS number[8].

Miscellaneous

Patients with obsessions constitute another group of difficult patients. Some have food fads. Others are preoccupied with diseases which can neither be proved or disproved. Others claim to have multiple allergies, or to react adversely to every drug they are given. Some patients are convinced that they are deficient in vitamins, or are being poisoned by lead in the domestic water supply, or are suffering from some obscure form of infection. The chronic fatigue syndrome, myalgic encephalomyelitis, and premenstrual tension are syndromes which can seldom be confirmed or excluded by current laboratory tests.

Some patients are classed as difficult because their principles do not allow them to accept some widely used and valuable treatment for themselves or their children. Parents who reject vaccination for their children are one example. Jehovah's Witnesses, with their rejection of blood transfusion, are another. In this connection, it has been reported that all adult members of the Society carry cards, which are renewed annually, clearly stating their refusal to accept blood transfusion (and their acceptance of possible non-blood alternatives such as Hartmann's solution), and releasing hospital staff from any liability for any untoward effects that might occur as a consequence of the prohibition[9]. Jehovah's Witnesses maintain a network of hospital liaison committees to assist in linking patients and doctors with specialists prepared to manage patients in harmony with their conscience[10].

Some patients are excessively demanding and uncooperative. They keep the doctor waiting or insist on ambulance transport unnecessarily. They complain unreasonably of being kept waiting themselves. They complain of the doctor's attitude. They refuse to be examined by students. They reject offers of home help or admission to an old people's home. Few actually go to the length of submitting written complaints, and many of those who do show clearly that they are mentally odd, often paranoid. In some illnesses, such as diabetes, the patient's cooperation is essential. If he is unwilling to cooperate, the doctor is in a 'no-win' situation.

The most unmanageable patient I have ever heard of was described in the *Journal of the Medical Defence Union*[11] in 1993. She was in her mid-20s, and her general practitioner recorded:

> *"This patient, allocated over the previous six months,*
> *has caused more practice disruption than all previous*
> *difficult patients put together. Her demands for*
> *medical attention have continued at a ridiculous*
> *frequency, and when the demands are refused she*
> *threatens (a) suicide (b) she will complain to the FHSA*
> *and allege assault. It is essential not to see her at home*
> *or in the surgery without a chaperone."*

There are hypochondriacs, like the invalid doctor who, after seeing top specialists in Edinburgh, sent elaborate diagrams of the site and radiation of his chest pain to a physician in Aberdeen, and sought his advice. There are lonely rich people who are bored, and who enjoy the notoriety of illness and the attention of a specialist.

Management of difficult patients

So far as the management of heart-sink patients is concerned, I have long considered that the only satisfactory approach is to review the notes comprehensively and summarise their contents. If this can be done in the presence of the patient so much the better, because he then sees the time and trouble the doctor is going through on his behalf. The doctor should attempt to view the problem from the patient's standpoint. Then he should state clearly what he can and cannot provide[12]. For the future, it should be arranged that, as far as possible, the patient should see the same doctor at each attendance.

Novack[13] makes the following practical points:

1. Reassurance that nothing is wrong does not help. The patient wants the physician to agree that he or she is sick.

2. Little is gained by a premature explanation that the symptoms are emotional.

3. The patient does not want symptom relief, but rather a relationship and understanding.

4. A positive organic diagnosis will not cure the patient.

5. Regular appointments are required so that the patient need not manifest symptoms to get help.

A centre has recently been opened in London specifically to provide treatment for heart-sink patients. It is multidisciplinary, with an emphasis on psychiatric expertise. It offers a flexible service. For some patients, assistance might be provided for assessment at their general practitioner's surgery. Others might require a four-to six-week assessment — as an inpatient if they live far from London — before a method of treatment could be proposed[14]. It is too soon to know whether this initiative will be successful, but it looks promising.

References

1. Hartnell L (1987) Personal view. *Br Med J* **294**:1029

2. Mayou R (1991) Medically unexplained physical symptoms. *Br Med J* **303**: 534–5

3. O'Dowd TC (1988) Five years of heart-sink patients in general practice. *Br Med J* **297**: 528–30

4. *Br J Medical Economics* (1992) quoted by *The Times* **24 July** 1992

5. Bayliss RIS (1984) The deceivers. *Br Med J* **288**: 583–4

6. Pallis CA, Bamji AN (1979) McIlroy was here, Or was he? *Br Med J* **i**: 973–5

7.   Spiers ASD (1993) Personal unique numbers (PUNS): their social potential. *Proc R Coll Physicians Edinb* 23: 239–45

8.   Tonks A (1993) Information management and patient privacy in the NHS. *Br Med J* 307: 1227–8

9.   Fry M (1994) Jehovah's Witnesses and the issue of blood transfusions. *J Christian Med Fellowship* 40: 2–6

10. Brace JWA (1992) Treating Jehovah's Witnesses (letter). *Br Med J* 305:

11. Medical Defence Union (1993) A most difficult patient. J *Med Defence Union* 9: 57–9

12. Jewell D (1988) I do not love thee Mr Fell. *Br Med J* 297: 498–9

13. Novack DH (1993) Active management of problem patients. *Brit J Hosp Med* 50: 573–4

14. Court C (1994) New day centre offers hope for "heart-sink" patients. *Br Med J* 309: 500

Chapter 11
TOTAL PATIENT CARE

◆ The importance of social and spiritual factors
◆ Why the consultant should be involved
◆ Examples of total patient care

The true role of the consultant goes beyond the physical and psychological needs of the patient to include the social and spiritual dimensions. To ignore these elements is to practise as a technician rather than a physician.

It is a remarkable fact that, at a time when medical science is advancing more rapidly than ever before, there is an unprecedented drift to unscientific healers whose ministrations are of no proven value. There are, no doubt, several reasons for this. One is undoubtedly a deep fear of the side-effects of the powerful drugs used in conventional medical treatment. But in my view, the main reason is that scientific medicine has lost the art of treating patients as people, consisting of body, mind and spirit. This is particularly a temptation for those specialists who deal with only a part of the patient.

This attitude derives from undergraduate teaching in which the doctor is taught to 'home in' on the specific area of physical or psychological pathology, identify it precisely and then attempt to correct it. But the truth is that matters are not always so simple. For many patients presenting with physical illness, social factors are vital. In others, there are what may be called 'spiritual' factors; examples include a sense of purposelessness, a feeling of guilt, or a fear of death. The fact is that most of the ills which afflict humans and cause them unhappiness are not susceptible to medical solutions. Balint[1] stated:

> "More often than scientific medicine cares to admit, it is not with a part but with the whole man that something has gone wrong, so that not one part but the whole man must be examined."

Prince Charles has repeatedly, and in my view rightly, criticised the medical profession for failing to treat 'the whole man'; for being unable to recognise *"sickness of the spirit"* — a *"sick soul disguised as an ailment of the body".*[2]

A problem the consultant cannot avoid

The consultant may argue that the social and spiritual needs of the patient are not his responsibility but those of the family doctor, who is traditionally the patient's guide, counsellor and friend. Many general practitioners, however, complain that with their increasingly busy schedule they are unable to undertake the care of the non-medical component of their patients' needs.

In any case, consultants have to face the fact that in many of the patients who are sent to them the basic problem is not physical or psychological, but spiritual. Such patients may present with a physical symptom purely to gain a hearing for their 'real' illness. This is well illustrated by the experience of Martyn Lloyd-Jones when he was working as medical registrar to Lord Horder. Horder asked him to prepare a diagnostic classification and analysis of his private patients. Lloyd-Jones[3] discovered that in well over 50% of cases the diagnosis was not a specific disease, but a comment such as *"eats too much"*, *"drinks too much"*, *"does not get enough sleep"* or *"is unhappy at home"*. This was one of the factors which led Lloyd-Jones eventually to leave medical practice and enter the full-time Christian ministry.

What does the consultant say to people who have no specific physical or psychological disease? Often, it must be admitted, he can only offer reassurance that there is nothing seriously wrong. He may be tempted to conclude that they really need a psychiatrist. But, in fact, these are not psychiatric problems, and some eminent psychiatrists have emphasised this fact. Jung[4] wrote:

> *"Among all my patients in the second half of life —*
> *that is to say over 35 — there has not been one whose*
> *problem in the last resort was not that of finding a*
> *religious outlook on life."*

A recent president of the Royal College of Psychiatrists used the occasion of his valedictory lecture to impress on his colleagues the importance of the spiritual dimension of their patients' lives[5].

The Department of Health acknowledges the spiritual needs of patients by supporting the appointment of hospital chaplains. It has recently reaffirmed its concern for this dimension of patient care by issuing a paper entitled *Meeting the Spiritual Needs of Patients and Staff: Good Practice Guidance*[6].

Whose job is it?

Granted that the patient's non-medical, and particularly his spiritual, needs are important, is it the hospital specialist's job to deal with them? Is it not the job for the minister of religion? In some cases, undoubtedly it is. Some hospitals are fortunate in having chaplains who are willing to help. But they can assist only a tiny minority, and in many cases their ministry is unacceptable to the patient.

In some specialties, problems of this nature are so common that every doctor should learn how to handle them. This is so in a children's oncology ward. A child undergoing inpatient treatment for leukaemia notices that another child receiving treatment similar to hers gets worse. Then, one morning the other child's bed is empty. She rightly concludes that she has died. So she asks the doctor or nurse, quite naturally, what will happen to her when she dies. The hospital staff cannot evade this question, much as they might wish to do so. It is not a problem for a psychiatrist or a chaplain. It is a medical problem.

It may be argued that there is a danger in encouraging doctors to express religious views to their patients. The General Medical Council[7], however, has made it clear that, although it is wrong for doctors to *"express personal beliefs in ways which may cause distress or which exploit patients' vulnerability"*, there is nothing to stop them expressing their personal religious (or, indeed, their political) views to patients. I would like to add three provisos. First, the doctor's comments must be relevant to the patient's perceived need. Second, they must be natural and not forced. Third, they should normally simply take the form of a sharing of personal experience. For instance, if a patient expresses a fear of surgery, the doctor might say: *"I would hate it too; but in such situations, I have found it a great help to commit my problem to God in prayer."*

Not a few of our patients actually have a tried and tested personal faith which enables them to face death calmly. I had the responsibility of looking after a former principal of Aberdeen University in his last illness. He had sustained a massive myocardial infarction. I saw him for the last time at four o'clock in the morning. He was in a state of cardiac shock: cold and clammy, but mentally alert. He gave me a calm smile. Two hours later, he was dead. Following the funeral, I received a letter from his widow, which included the following sentence (which I quote with her permission): *"I think you will like to know that almost his last words were: 'If my Lord calls me now, I am ready to come.'"* Such words, uttered to one's closest companion within minutes of the end of life, are likely to be real.

Dealing with guilt

For many patients, the underlying problem is a sense of guilt. Sometimes, the feeling of guilt is inappropriate, and based on a misunderstanding. If this can be resolved, the benefit may be tremendous. In other cases, a sense of guilt is entirely appropriate. A gynaecologist friend of mine was consulted by a patient with urinary symptoms. He was impressed by her miserable appearance and said to her: *"You are an unhappy woman. Would you like to tell me about it?"* After some hesitation, she proceeded to confess that she had smothered her mother, and could not get it out of her mind.

This is an extreme example, but a burden of guilt is much more common than we often realise. Many patients recovering from a road traffic accident are burdened by self-accusation as they recall that injuries sustained by others were the result of their carelessness. A sense of guilt is common among patients undergoing termination of pregnancy. A hospital chaplain found one of them in tears. When he asked her what was wrong, she replied: *"I'm a murderer."*

Awareness of actual guilt (as distinct from mere guilt feelings) may hinder a patient's response to treatment. Tournier[8] gave an example of this from his experience. He had under his care a medical colleague in whom a minor local infection had developed into septicaemia. This illness responded surprisingly badly to treatment. The patient had to remain in hospital for several months and was left with a lasting feeling of exhaustion. Eventually, he resolved to speak frankly to his physician. He told him how a 'lapse' as a student had led to financial difficulties, about which he had never spoken to his wife, and which had led to him using her money to meet his debts. He was hoping to extricate himself by taking on a heavier work-load, but he never succeeded in getting out of debt. Tournier made two diagnoses in this case The first was a physical one: septicaemia. The other was a spiritual one: guilt. Once the patient accepted this double diagnosis, he recovered rapidly and completely.

Total patient care in practice

Early in my medical career, I had a remarkable experience of the therapeutic effect of a personal Christian faith. A doctor was admitted to my ward with inoperable carcinoma of the stomach. He was too ill to send home, and I did not have a single room for him, so he had to share a two-bedded room with a young man recently returned from India, whom I was investigating for amoebic dysentery. It so happened that this young man had had an experience of Christian conversion, and his quiet peace of mind was a good advertisement for the faith. At first the old doctor was bitter and resentful at his fate, and I recoiled at the prospect of my daily visit to him. After a week or so, however, his attitude completely changed. I found that the old doctor had found peace with God.

Solomon Papper[9] summed up the role of the consultant as *"deep concern for and commitment to the patient and his physical, psychological, social and spiritual life."* If the specialist is to attempt to fill this demanding role, he must show himself to be open to comments and questions which are not strictly related to his specialty. This is difficult under NHS conditions for, although the Department of Health acknowledges the spiritual needs of patients, the volume of work demanded from doctors and nurses is such that the spiritual dimension is virtually squeezed out. It is easier in private practice, where the specialist can set his own agenda, and plan the ambience of his consulting suite appropriately. For example, I used to display in my waiting room a framed verse from the Bible stating: *"All things work together for good to them that love God."*

Even in NHS practice, where there's a will, there's a way. A surgeon of my acquaintance used to send each patient admitted to hospital under his care a personal signed letter with an invitation to approach him regarding any personal needs. The letter ended:

> *"Please be assured you are not just a 'case'. You are a*
> *person with needs of body and mind and spirit and*
> *you live in a home perhaps beset with many problems.*
> *I hope you will go from here better equipped to deal*
> *with life and with all its demands and perplexities."*

That was an attempt to treat the whole patient.

Conclusion

The concept of holistic medicine is often ridiculed by pointing out that when a patient is 'really ill' he needs, not a wise father-figure but the best specialist in the relevant field. This may be true in the case of patients with acute illnesses or gross lesions. But in the great majority of those seen in consulting practice, a whole patient approach is needed; treating patients as people, finding out about their way of life, their interests, and what makes them tick — although always respecting their reticence. Rightly handled, this has the advantage that the patient develops confidence in his physician with consequent improved compliance and therapeutic benefit.

References

1. Balint M (1965) The doctor's therapeutic function. *Lancet* **i**: 1177–80

2. The Prince of Wales (1982) A personal message. *Br Med J* **285**: 1

3. Lloyd-Jones M (1982) *The Doctor Himself.* Christian Medical Fellowship, London: 23

4. Jung C (1933) *Modern Man in Search of a Soul.* Kegan Paul, London: 264

5. Sims A (1994) 'Psyche' — Spirit as well as Mind? *Br J Psych* **165**: 441–6

6. Department of Health Annex (1992) Meeting the spiritual needs of patients and staff: good practice guidance. *HSG*, **92**: 2

7. General Medical Council (1993) *Br Med J* **307**: 1286

8. Tournier P (1954) *A Doctor's Case Book.* SCM.Press, London: 11–16

9. Papper S (1983) *Doing Right.* Little, Brown and Co, Boston: 20

Chapter 12
LEARNING FROM OUR MISTAKES

◆ The high frequency of medical mistakes
◆ Non-negligent mistakes
◆ Mistakes in diagnosis
◆ Mistakes in management
◆ Reasons for mistakes
◆ Learning from mistakes

Doctors' mistakes are, unfortunately, frequently in the news and make irresistible reading. Every doctor, however experienced and conscientious, makes mistakes, some of which have serious results. Our natural inclination is to try to conceal them and forget about them. But McIntyre and Popper[1] have urged that we should make a determined effort to recognise them and learn from them. They have gone so far as to claim that knowledge grows more by the recognition of errors than by the accumulation of facts, so that, in their view, learning from our mistakes should take precedence over the acquisition of new information.

Frequency of medical mistakes

It is impossible to determine the frequency of medical mistakes but there can be no doubt that they are much more common than most of us realise. The protection societies have information on the annual rate of claims and complaints but this is only a fraction of the total number of accidents. The only published information currently available comes from the USA. A study conducted in California in 1974 concluded that 3 million hospital admissions led to 140 000 injuries, an incidence of 4.7%[2]. A more recent review[3], conducted in New York State, concluded that 2.7 million hospital admissions led to 98 600 adverse events; an incidence of 3.7%. With five million hospital admissions a year in England alone, this might mean almost 200 000 medical accidents in English hospitals.

Many accidents never come to light, because the outcome was not unexpected. Thus, delay in the diagnosis of cancer or diabetes may remain unsuspected by the patient or his relatives. In many cases, only the doctor at fault, and perhaps one or two others, know that there was a mistake. There are many relatively minor errors which have no serious consequence. Risky practices only occasionally lead to disaster. A doctor may go off duty early and be out of contact with the hospital or with his patients. The fact will only come to light if there is some sudden, fatal complication, such as a pulmonary embolism.

Mistakes do not necessarily indicate negligence

Most medical accidents are due, in some degree, to error, even if it is only a failure of anticipation. But most errors do not involve actual negligence[4]. For example, an obstetrician concluded, after careful examination, that the breech baby was too big to be delivered safely by the vaginal route, so he decided to do a caesarean section. At operation, he found that the baby was in fact quite small and could safely have been delivered naturally. The mother had a healthy baby, so she did not question the obstetrician's decision. Nevertheless, she was put at additional risk and was left with a scar in her uterus. In the event, her next pregnancy ended in uterine rupture and death of her full-term baby. The obstetrician made an error of judgement, but he could not be called negligent.

Conscientious doctors make mistakes through ignorance or inexperience. In the study from California, quoted above, only one in six of the injuries were classified as being due to negligence, in the study from New York State, less than a quarter.

The General Medical Council recognises three levels of misdemeanour by doctors. The first is serious medical misconduct. The second is the situation in which competence is seriously impaired by sickness, often due to misuse of alcohol or drugs. The third is unacceptable behaviour, for example, rudeness, or systematic lateness for clinics. Most medical mistakes, however, do not qualify for consideration by the General Medical Council.

Mistakes in diagnosis

Doctors make mistakes in diagnosis, treatment and prognosis. The most important mistakes are those in which the diagnosis of a serious disease was missed or in which the wrong treatment was applied. If the disease is acute, the mistake may be rapidly fatal. Fortunately, this is not often the case. More often, the doctor has an opportunity to revise his diagnosis and apply the correct treatment in time to avoid permanent damage.

Diagnosis may be delayed because the significance of the signs and symptoms is not appreciated when the patient is first seen. When this happens in a patient with cancer, the possibility of cure may be lost. Sometimes a diagnosis is delayed or overlooked because, although the essential information for making a correct diagnosis was available, a key report remained unread or unappreciated. This applies particularly to radiologists' reports and reports on cervical smears.

Mistakes in management

The wrong treatment may be given through ignorance or carelessness. Some mistakes simply reflect the ignorance of the day. Fifty years ago, it was widely accepted that premature infants should be treated with high concentrations of oxygen. Now it is recognised that such treatment contributes to retinopathy. The history of medicine is littered with discarded treatments.

In the past, patients have been entered for research projects without their consent. Most came to no harm, but a few were injured as a result. Since this misconduct was exposed and ethical committees were established in all medical institutions, this practice has become much rarer. It would, however, be unduly optimistic to say that it has been completely eliminated.

Prognosis is never certain and every doctor makes mistakes in attempting to forecast the outcome of disease, particularly at an early stage in his career. Sometimes I failed to appreciate the seriousness of a patient's condition. More often I took an unduly pessimistic view, although usually without indicating this to the patient.

Reasons for mistakes

The commonest reasons for medical mistakes are ignorance, errors of judgement and carelessness. Ignorance is, to some extent, inevitable. Even the most erudite and experienced doctors have large gaps in their medical knowledge. Knowledge is advancing so rapidly that no doctor can know everything, even in his own specialty.

Many mistakes are due to inexperience. The doctor may have up-to-date book knowledge but may never have actually seen some of the important diseases that he is called upon to treat. The circumstances may be such that he is compelled to undertake a risky procedure without supervision. Or he may be a well-informed specialist in one branch of medicine, but with little experience in another disease which affects his patient. Some doctors are adventurers and are happy to attempt techniques in which they are inexperienced, without adequate supervision.

Errors of judgement are also inevitable. Medical diagnosis and treatment is not an exact science. There are always a number of imponderables in every situation. The results of investigations may be misleading. Every patient acts and reacts differently. Experience helps, but even the most experienced doctor is liable to misjudge a situation.

Occasional carelessness is universal, since doctors are human. Carelessness, in the broadest sense, is probably an important factor in medical mistakes. There is a good deal of truth in the saying: *"More mistakes are made through not caring than through not knowing."* There is a tendency in all of us to put personal comfort before patient care. This was memorably highlighted in an anonymous article in *The Lancet*[5], under the title: *"The man who never comes back."* All doctors are, at times, distracted by family or business matters. Some are constitutionally more considerate, careful and obsessional than others.

No consideration of reasons for medical mistakes would be complete without mention of organisational and environmental factors. These are undoubtedly important. Doctors make more mistakes when they are tired and rushed, because there is then a tendency to cut corners. Where such a situation exists, doctors have a duty, both to themselves and to the service, to make joint representation to those responsible for management. On the other hand, we must resist the temptation to put all the blame for our mistakes on 'the system'.

Avoidance of mistakes

Every doctor should make it a matter of honour to keep abreast of the advances in medical knowledge in his specialty and also in the major advances in other specialties. The importance of continuing medical education is now widely recognised and this method keeping up-to-date is likely to become compulsory before long. Ideally, a doctor should not undertake any work for which he is not equipped or in which he has not an experienced colleague to consult. This is, of course, a counsel of perfection, because in real life there are some situations in which a doctor finds himself out of his depth through unforeseen circumstances. He has no-one to turn to and simply has to do the best he can.

An important way in which doctors can avoid mistakes and learn to correct their individual bias is by consultation with colleagues. One of the most valuable correctives for me, as a cardiologist, was the departmental combined cardiac clinic. At this clinic, my physician colleagues and I met with a cardiac surgeon and a radiologist, as well as with our junior staff, to pool our ideas about the diagnosis and treatment of the more complex problems we had encountered. Another educational practice which I adopted was attendance on the ward rounds of other consultants, by prior arrangement.

Learning from mistakes

If McIntyre and Popper[1] are right, and knowledge grows supremely from the recognition of errors, how, in practice, can we do this? Obviously, we need to keep good records and do our best to follow up our problem patients. Without accurate records, it is impossible to know how often we are mistaken in our original diagnoses. Early in my consultant career, I opened a file entitled 'Diagnostic puzzles' for cases in which I could not reach a diagnosis. By going through this file periodically, it was interesting to find that time had solved some of them, with consequent educational benefit. It is valuable to keep a note of our mistakes in the same way that Darwin kept a note of facts which appeared to conflict with his theories.

We need help and cooperation in discovering and analysing our errors, and that is where peer review audit is invaluable. Doctors generally are very reluctant to admit to others that they make mistakes. When I initiated an audit session for the Division of Medicine, it was not well attended. Not surprisingly, it was the most conscientious and respected doctors who made time for the exercise. Criticism should, of course, be constructive and there must be a willingness to accept it. It should be a rule that all those who attend should, from time to time, have their cases reviewed. There should be no mere spectators. On the other hand, involving outsiders is valuable if they approach problems from a different background.

Negative criticism should be excluded. If there is a fear of being shown up — of being made the scapegoat or of appearing ignorant or looking foolish — the exercise is doomed to failure. No-one likes being shown up as having made a mistake, and doctors are only human. In our case, however, there is an additional consideration: the fear that if our patients found out that we made mistakes, it would undermine their confidence in us. Patients prefer the illusion that although some doctors make mistakes, their own doctor is infallible, or nearly so!

In addition to peer review audit, doctors should consult with other members of the caring team. For example, it would be good for doctors to ask senior ward and outpatient nursing staff: *"Can you suggest a better way of running the clinic?"* or *"Is there anything I could have done last week that would have made your work easier?"*

We can also learn much by comparing British practice with that of other advanced countries, where this differs markedly from our own. There are, in fact, large and unexplained variations in medical practice between Britain, France, Germany, Scandinavia and North America[6]. This is particularly true of the management of caesarean section, breast cancer, prostate disease, coronary angiography, upper gastrointestinal endoscopy, carotid endarterectomy, cholesterol testing and, especially, hysterectomy, which shows a seven-fold variation between Norway and the USA. Some, at least, of these differences must reflect uncertainty regarding the best treatment.

Even within one country, there is wide variation in practice in relation to some conditions. For example, in a study of ENT practice, it was found that one specialist recommended tonsillectomy for 50% of the patients referred to him. It was arranged that those who were not advised surgery should be sent to another ENT surgeon. He recommended surgery for 50% of these. Those for whom he did not advise surgery were sent to a third ENT specialist, who recommended surgery on 50% of those rejected by the two previous surgeons. There must surely be something to learn here.

Overtreatment is both wasteful and risky, and inevitably denies resources to others. We must face the challenge of practice variation, otherwise we shall be vulnerable to government criticism that we are misapplying resources. If we do not regulate our own practice, it will be done from outside the profession, and be dictated more by economic than by quality considerations.

Doctors, however experienced and eminent, can never sit back and rest on their laurels. They must constantly be reading and sharing their experiences with their colleagues. As Lord Lister is reported to have said: *"If you are not willing to learn and unlearn all your life through, you should give up medicine and take up a third-rate trade."*

References

1. McIntyre N, Popper K (1983) The critical attitude in medicine: the need for a new ethics. *Br Med J* **287**: 1919–24

2. Smith R (1986) When things go wrong. *Br Med J* **293**: 461–2

3. Harvard Medical Practice Study (1990) *Patients, Doctors and Lawyers; Medical Injury, Malpractice Litigation and Patient Compensation in New York.* Harvard Medical Practice Study, Boston

4. Vincent CA (1989) Research into medical accidents: a case of negligence? *Br Med J* **299**: 1150–3

5. *Lancet* (1979) The man who never comes back. *Lancet,* **ii**: 1358–9

6. Anderson TF, Mooney G (1990) *The Challenge of Medical Practice Variations.* Macmillan Press, London

Chapter 13
TEAM CARE

- ◆ The inevitability of shared care
- ◆ Its disadvantages
- ◆ Its advantages
- ◆ Striking a balance
- ◆ Consultant clinics in general practitioner health centres

In all developed countries, team care is one of the facts of life. In British medical practice, the general practitioner is, so far as the patient is concerned, the head of the team, and the specialist his expert assistant brought in to advise on a specific aspect of medical care. It is important for the consultant to appreciate this. The general practitioner knows the patient and his circumstances better than the specialist, and the general practitioner has to retain the patient's confidence in a continuing way long after the 'incident' of the specialist consultation has become a thing of the past. All major recommendations to the patient should therefore be channelled through the general practitioner.

Although my primary concern in this chapter is the team of doctors, it is important to recognise that the team concept extends far beyond this central core. It embraces everyone whose activities impinge on the patient's welfare including the receptionist, the nurses, the physiotherapists, the dietician, the porters and ambulance staff to the 'back-room' radiologists and laboratory technicians whom the patient never sees. Any plan for improving the service to the patient must embrace the wider team concept, otherwise it is doomed to failure.

The situation in hospital clinics

The hospital consultant is the head of the hospital team, and the patients who pass through his clinics and wards are administratively under his care. In practice, he may see some of them for only a few minutes, or not at all. In a study of 4275 outpatient consultations in a district general hospital, it was found that less than half of the new surgical patients and only one-third of all surgical patients attending the clinic were seen by a consultant. Nine months later, about one-third of all new patients had still not seen a consultant in the clinic. In the medical clinics, one-quarter of the patients were seen by doctors who had had less than six months' experience in their present specialty after registration[1]. Another study, analysing 288 referrals to orthopaedic departments in teaching hospitals, showed that whereas the referral letter was almost always written by a principal in general practice, the reply was written by the consultant in only half the cases. The remainder were written by a senior registrar or a registrar, or occasionally by a senior house officer[2].

Such a delegation of the outpatient workload is traditional in almost all departments. It is justified on two grounds: first, that there are not enough consultants to see all the patients referred to the outpatient clinic and second, that junior doctors have to learn by being given responsibility.

The existence of team care means that there is no assurance that at review appointments the patient will see the same doctor as on the previous occasion. It is not surprising, therefore, that the two commonest complaints made about specialist outpatient clinics are *"I didn't see the consultant"* and, in the case of patients attending for follow-up *"I never see the same doctor twice"*.

This situation is not peculiar to hospital practice. A similar 'merry-go-round' is seen in general practice. A survey of three large group practices with combined lists showed that of consultations with patients who had attended the health centre on 12 occasions, only about half had been with the same doctor. In one practice more than a quarter of the patients had consulted seven or more doctors, and one-tenth had consulted nine or ten. Many of these doctors were trainees and locums. In the case of children, it was even worse. Sixty-three out of 72 children consulted at least five doctors over 12 consecutive attendances[3].

A few consultants arrange to see all patients referred to them, but this inevitably restricts the number of patients who can be seen at their clinics. The present situation cannot improve until there is a radical change in the balance between consultants and junior staff.

Disadvantages of team care

Most patients feel that the present state of affairs is unsatisfactory. As one of them put it: *"Seeing different staff at each hospital visit is disorientating and alienating."* Continuity is essential if patients are to have a chance to understand and participate in health care encounters. Patients rate highly the relationship with the individual doctor. They like to be able to speak of *"My doctor."* Furthermore, they prefer that this key figure is the first person to whom they pour out their story[4].

> *"When a person once unburdens himself to a confidant (which in itself often requires a considerable amount of moral courage) he does not want to repeat his story all over again to someone else. The important time is the first time the patient speaks."*[5]

Seeing a different doctor on repeated visits is not merely perceived by the patient as being unsatisfactory, it has definite disadvantages so far as his management is concerned. In the first place, the second doctor cannot be aware of all the facts which are in the first doctor's possession. There are many facts about patients which it is impossible to record in the notes. This applies particularly to the most sensitive information. Team care is disadvantageous so far as the deeper, psychological needs of the patient are concerned. These can only be understood and dealt with on a one-to-one basis. An inevitable result of seeing more than one doctor is embarrassment and sometimes conflicting advice. In addition, the patient is presented with an irresistible temptation to play one doctor off against another. Personal, continuous care is linked with patient satisfaction. If patient satisfaction is accepted as an integral part of quality health care, reinforcing personal care may be one way of increasing this quality. There is no doubt that a multiplicity of doctors occasionally results in serious mismanagement[6].

It is difficult for a junior doctor who is seeing a patient only once to feel a full sense of responsibility when a diagnosis has already been made and treatment has commenced. If the doctor is in a hurry, he will not trouble to go through all the notes, but simply do the minimum necessary and give the patient a fresh appointment, hoping that it will be someone else's problem next time. Most junior doctors are reluctant to discharge patients from outpatient follow-up.

This state of affairs is, of course, unsatisfactory, not only for the patient but also for the referring doctor. It is the advice of the consultant he wants, not that of the trainee.

Advantages of team care

All is not loss, however. Indeed, it has been argued that the needs of patients are, in practice, best met by a plurality of doctors — specifically by 'a team of three'[7]. In the first place, the patient needs a doctor who is constantly available. In hospital this must, perforce, be a junior doctor. Secondly, he wants, and often needs, the most up-to-date medicine available. This is supplied by a registrar. Thirdly, he wants a doctor with experience. This need is supplied by the consultant. Junior staff and even medical students sometimes contribute a fresh and up-to-date viewpoint. After all, some of them will in future be leaders of the profession. We all know of instances in which the locum has had the flash of inspiration which has eluded the more experienced regular doctor.

Team care also goes some way towards ensuring that patients are not at the mercy of an individual doctor with cranky ideas.

In any case, team work is unavoidable. Every doctor has to take holidays and attend conferences to keep up to date. No doctor can be available for every emergency in his patients. Moreover, students and postgraduates have to learn how to manage patients, and there is no effective substitute for learning on the job. Now that the trend is increasingly towards avoiding admission to hospital whenever possible, more investigations are being done in the outpatient department; so that outpatient training is likely to increase rather than decrease.

Striking a balance

How can the ideal of a personal doctor for each patient be attained or approached? There is no perfect solution. One model is for the most experienced doctor to make the decisions, with input from his bright young colleagues, and their assistance with special procedures within their capabilities and under his instruction. I saw what I still consider an excellent system when I sat in on a clinic at the Hospital for Sick Children, in Great Ormond Street, in the 1960s. The consultant took the history, flanked by three or four assistants. Then he sent one of the assistants off with the mother and her child to conduct the examination and report back to him. The consultant then checked any positive findings, made the final decision and spoke to the mother.

I have never seen this procedure in action anywhere else. When I attempted it, I quickly sensed that my junior staff, who had been brought up on a different system, regarded it as too hierarchical and 'bossy'. They preferred to be in complete charge of any patient they saw, asking the consultant's advice at their discretion. Any system in which the consultant sees all the patients inevitably means that fewer patients can be seen in a given period of time, thus increasing the waiting time for outpatient appointments. Another disadvantage of the above system is that the patient does not see the consultant on his own.

A compromise solution which has been suggested is for the new patients to be shared between the consultant and his more experienced junior staff, with all review patients being seen by the consultant at every third or fourth attendance, or if the junior doctor is absent. This would provide junior staff with experience in assessing new patients, ensure exchange of information between senior and junior staff, allow the consultant to pursue a vigorous policy of discharge, and avoid the complaint that patients never see the same doctor twice[8]. Another system is for the consultant to see all the new patients, leaving the juniors to do the follow-ups. This goes some way towards satisfying the general practitioners but does nothing to avoid the patient's disappointment at seeing different doctors on subsequent occasions.

The limited number of consultants is the great problem. Every patient naturally wants to see the specialist, and every general practitioner wants the specialist to see his patient. This could only be achieved by a considerable expansion in consultant staffing — much greater than is currently envisaged.

It is important that the consultant should give due recognition to his team by showing them consideration and not overworking them, by acknowledging their contribution, by communicating freely with them and bringing them into the decision-making process whenever possible, and by backing them up when things go wrong.

Consultant clinics in general practitioner health centres

There has recently been increased interest in consultants carrying out clinics in general practitioner health centres. There are obvious advantages to the patients, to the general practitioners and to the consultants. The patients are on more familiar ground, and have the opportunity of face-to-face discussion with the general practitioner and the consultant together. The general practitioners get to know the consultant personally and can discuss other patients with him. For the consultant, there is something nearer to a private consultation than is possible in most hospitals. There are, of course, disadvantages, particularly the lack of the full range of skills of specialist nurses and the investigation facilities of the main hospital[9]. This form of consultation is not universally applicable but appears to have worked satisfactorily in dermatology, ophthalmology, orthopaedics and ENT. The fear has, however, been expressed that the growth of outreach clinics may gradually but inexorably provide open access to patients without the need for referral. If self-referral became widespread, it would undermine the general practitioner's responsibility to unravel the patient's symptoms, and help him choose discriminately when specialist advice is needed[10].

References

1.   Kiff RS, Sykes PA (1988) Who undertakes the consultations in the outpatient department? *Br Med J* **296**: 1511–12

2.   Jacobs LGH, Pringle MA (1990) Referral letters and replies from orthopaedic departments: opportunities missed. *Br Med J* **301**: 470–3

3.   Freeman GK, Richards SC (1990) How much personal care in four group practices? *Br Med J* **301**: 1028–30

4.   Boyd WD (1987) Talking to patients — the problems. *Proc R Coll Physicians Edinb* **17**: 173–84

5.   Hunt JH (1969) Religion and the family doctor. *Proc R Soc Med* **62**: 341–6

6.   Medical Defence Union (1989) *Annual Report*: 18–19

7.   Browse N (1981) In defence of the team of three. *World Med* **(Feb 21st)**: 47

8.   Fowler AW (1988) Outpatient consultations (letter). *Br Med J* **297**: 293

9.   Collins CD (1994) Advantages of consultant clinics in GP practices (letter). *Brit J Hosp Med* **51**: 377

10.   Sweeney B (1994) The referral system. *Br Med J* **309**: 1180–1

Chapter 14
PITFALLS IN THE CONSULTANT'S PATH

- ◆ The importance of maintaining the profession's reputation
- ◆ Greed
- ◆ Dishonesty
- ◆ Arrogance
- ◆ Alcohol and drug abuse
- ◆ Neglect of wife and family
- ◆ Neglect of recreation

If the consultant is to retain his skill and his reputation, he must be constantly aware of the pitfalls that lie in his path.

Maintaining the trust of the public

The success of medical consultation depends largely on trust between patient and doctor. The basis of this trust is the reputation, both of the individual doctor and also of the profession as a whole. What can happen if a profession forfeits the trust of the public is well illustrated by the sharp decline in the reputation of the police force in Britain during the second half of the 20th century. A generation ago, the police were generally respected and admired. Now, following a series of revelations of dishonesty leading to miscarriages of justice, they are widely distrusted. Moreover, this attitude of distrust inevitably affects the work of the individual member of the force, with the result that a policeman making an arrest can no longer expect the same support from the public as in the past.

Precisely the same consideration applies to the medical profession. Adverse publicity regarding individual doctors inevitably leads to a lessened regard for the profession as a whole;

this in turn affects, to some degree, every consultation. We are fortunate to be practising in an era when the reputation of doctors, in Britain at least, has for decades been higher than that of any other profession. But it has not always been so. Before the 18th century, the standing of doctors in Britain was low — surgeons were classed with barbers, and doctors would normally go to the servants' entrance of a great house — and this low reputation persisted to the end of the 19th century[1].

The present high esteem in which the profession is held cannot be taken for granted. It has been painstakingly gained by a combination of wise leadership, successful scientific research and a reputation for integrity. Advances in treatment do not, in themselves, ensure respect. Unless they are combined with wisdom and compassion they may just as easily breed fear. So the regard in which the profession is held must be carefully cherished. Every doctor has a responsibility to future generations to maintain and, if possible, enhance the reputation of the profession. There is some evidence that the standing of doctors in the USA has fallen perceptibly during recent decades[2] with a corresponding rise in litigation against them. The same could happen here.

Greed

The decline in respect for the medical profession in the USA has been associated with what is perceived as the growing commercialisation of medicine. Although consultants in the Western world are well paid, this is no protection against the sin of greed. A perception that doctors are greedy for money is undoubtedly a frequent criticism of the profession. The amusing notice on the back of the door of one of our medical deans has an element of truth: *"Money isn't everything — but it is a long way ahead of whatever is in second place."* Doctors are known to be among the most highly paid members of society, so that evidence of greed appears inexcusable.

Greed may express itself in various forms. The doctor may make false claims for services undertaken, or initiate unnecessary investigations or treatment for which he can claim additional payment. Pharmaceutical companies are only too happy to invest money in doctors, in the hope of a good return in the form of an increased sale of their products.

In some of the less affluent countries, doctors are poorly paid, and many have succumbed to the temptation to demand bribes for services such as vasectomy or the fitting of an intrauterine coil, services which are part of the doctor's contract and should be free to the patient. There have also been many reliable reports of doctors demanding large sums of money before relieving a patient with retention of urine or undertaking emergency surgery.

The grosser forms of 'bribery' may not exist in Britain, nevertheless the temptation exists. Grateful patients and organisations offer money for research and equipment; this has been known to disappear into personal research funds, and thence into personal accounts. When this is discovered and publicised, not only is the individual doctor disgraced but the reputation of the profession is also besmirched. Not long ago, a gynaecologist was convicted of cheating the health service by booking a woman into an NHS hospital bed without disclosing that she was his private patient. He was jailed for 15 months. The saying *"A good name is more important than riches"* (Proverbs 22;1) is particularly true of medical consulting practice. *"Do not wear yourself out to get rich; have the wisdom to show restraint"* (Proverbs 23;4) is another piece of good advice.

Dishonesty

Dishonesty is closely linked with greed. Richard Cabot[3], an eminent American physician and medical statesman, in his book entitled *Honesty*, expressed himself amazed at the degree of acquiescence in dishonesty among medical practitioners in his day. His chief concern was the lies that doctors told their patients. He emphasised that one doctor's deceit undermined the patient's trust in the profession as a whole. Cabot conceded that honesty is easier for the older doctor. It is certainly easier for a doctor with an established reputation to confess his ignorance.

There is a temptation to abuse the trust of our patients.

Evidence of patients being entered into research projects without their knowledge and agreement casts a serious slur on the profession. Some reports of 'human guinea pigs' in the past[4] are almost incredible. But the lure of research is such that continual self-discipline and vigilance are needed. A medical secretary lost her faith in doctors when she had to type a paper which described how doctors sigmoidoscoped patients under anaesthesia without their permission in order to gain experience. There is also the temptation to treat patients with 'interesting' diseases beyond one's sphere of competence.

Arrogance

The modern doctor may not enjoy the privileges of his predecessors: a chauffeur-driven car; the head porter of the hospital standing at the door to take his hat and coat; the ward sister and the junior doctors awaiting him at the entrance to the ward. Nevertheless, he still has temptations enough to engender inflated ideas of his importance. This can easily lead to an attitude of arrogance toward his patients, and dominance over his assistants[5]. A general practitioner who spent part of his sabbatical leave attending hospital outpatient sessions was struck by the fact that a considerable number of consultants were habitually late, habitually had other commitments which always overran, or habitually allowed the gross overbooking of clinics so that the average time for consultations was reduced to a few minutes[6].

Alcohol and drug abuse

The commonest type of case considered by the Preliminary Proceedings Committee of the General Medical Council falls under the heading 'Disregard of professional responsibility to patients'. High on the list in this category comes abuse of alcohol and drugs. The temptation to abuse alcohol and drugs is strong in the medical profession. The doctor's life is stressful and drugs are easily obtainable. So the doctor is readily drawn towards these agents as a means of relaxation or stimulation. At first, their use is occasional, but gradually it becomes more frequent, until it leads to impairment of medical performance and ultimately, in some cases, to criminal negligence and ruinous publicity. It is probably true to say that more medical careers have been ruined by alcohol than by any other means[7].

Improper sexual behaviour

This is one of the major grounds for complaint to the General Medical Council regarding the behaviour of doctors. A fundamental principle of doctor/patient relationship is that the doctor will never exploit the patient's trust to gratify his or her own emotional, financial or sexual needs. And because the boundaries are defined by society, a patient can never be seen as giving valid consent for sexual activity. Such activity between physician and patient can never be justified on the grounds that the patient consented or even, on occasion, asked for or demanded it[8]. Any betrayal of trust leaves harmful legacies and impairs all future relationships. In view of the danger of temptation or of false accusation, there is much to be said for both male and female doctors habitually employing a chaperone[9].

In seeking sexual gratification outside marriage, doctors have to consider whether, in addition to wrecking their marriage, they may also be running a risk of human immunodeficiency virus (HIV) infection, with consequent damage to health and practice.

Neglect of wife and family

The most widespread and insidious temptation for the ambitious consultant is the neglect of wife and family. He comes home tired, and just wants to be left alone with the newspaper and the television. He has spent his day striving against major illness, and the last thing he wants is to have to show his ignorance regarding the treatment of a crying child of his own with an acute attack of earache or some other 'trivial' condition. By neglecting domestic responsibilities, husband and wife inevitably drift apart, and the doctor loses the vitally important stability of a calm and happy home life. Sir David Llewellyn MP gave sound advice when he said, in an open letter to a new member of Parliament:

> *"No matter what success you will have achieved, if*
> *your progress has been bought at the price of family,*
> *children, friends — or conscience — it will turn to dust*
> *and ashes in your mouth."*

Disraeli is reported as saying:

> *" A female friend, amiable, clever and devoted, is a*
> *possession more valuable than parks or palaces; and*
> *without such a Muse few men can succeed, and none*
> *can be happy."*

Frequently, the doctor's family suffers too. Here is part of a letter reportedly written by a consultant's daughter to her father[5].

"Dear Dad,

Lots of people have told me you are a great man. I believe that. I remember seeing your name in the paper a lot when I was growing up. ... And you never forgot a birthday. I remember I always received an airmail special delivery from somewhere back East. But how I longed for you to come home and share my day with me. You were up so early and came home when we were all in bed.

Yes you've given me a lot, dad, and I appreciate it. I'm educated. I'm well travelled. I know about music and art. But I wish you had had the time to really know me; because all I have are the newspaper clippings and the awards and the pictures. I really don't know you at all.

Your loving daughter"

Neglect of recreation

The doctor's life can easily become hopelessly unbalanced and, as a result, a poor example to his patients and to society generally. There is no doubt that the life of many doctors is dominated by work to a pathological degree. They come to like the 'image' of always being busy, always on call, important, essential. There is the constant temptation to take on more and more commitments: another committee, another hospital appointment, a research project or the writing of a review article. I have been amazed when doctors, who are already doing more than a full-time job, voluntarily take on additional work which could be done equally well by someone else.

Every worker, especially one who carries heavy responsibility, needs regular periods of rest and relaxation. Fatigue is apt to pass unnoticed, yet it insidiously undermines efficiency[10]. We all give good advice to our over-busy patients about the need for relaxation, yet we often break the rules ourselves. A wise old general practitioner colleague of mine used to quote the adage: "It is never a waste of time to stop to sharpen the scythe."

There is a widespread tendency for doctors to neglect their cultural and spiritual health. One doctor wrote to the British Medical Journal[11] a year after retirement:

> *"I found that I had been culturally and intellectually starved, even by so broad a subject as medicine. I was ignorant of any literature other than medical literature."*

If the consultant is to be the best practitioner and the best example to society, he needs to cultivate a balanced life — including the four ingredients which Cabot designated, namely work, play, love and worship[12].

Most consultants work right through to retirement without their conduct raising any serious concern among either their colleagues or among the public. A significant minority, however, do cause concern. A doctor involved in NHS administration found that the conduct of 6% of 850 senior medical staff in his area gave rise to consideration of disciplinary action[13]. The problems included poor attitude and disruptive or irresponsible behaviour (32 instances), lack of commitment to duties (21 instances), poor skills and inadequate knowledge (19 instances), dishonesty (11 instances), and sexual matters (7 instances).

References

1. Charles J (1954) The doctor's place in the community: some historical sidelights. *Lancet* **i**: 455–9

2. Blendon RJ (1988) The public's view of the future of health care. *JAMA* **259**: 3587–93

3. Cabot R (1938) *Honesty*. Macmillan Co, New York

4. Pappworth MH (1967) *Human Guinea Pigs*. Routledge and Kegan Paul, London

5. Kraybill DB, Good PP (1982) *Perils of Professionalism*. Herald Press, Ontario: 51–78

6. Cubitt T (1993) Crying out for succour (Personal View). *Br Med J* **306**: 800

7. Rawnsley K (1991) The national counselling service for sick doctors. *Proc R Coll Physicians Edinb* **21**: 4–7

8. Patterson PGR, Blackshaw S (1993) Abuse of patients by physicians. *Med N Am*, **October**: 721–4

9. Speelman A, Savage J, Verburgh M (1993) Use of chaperones by general practitioners. *Br Med J* **307**: 986–7

10. Douthwaite AH (1956) Pitfalls in medicine. *Br Med J* **ii**: 896–900

11. Thompson MK (1987) Retiring (letter). *Br Med J* **294**: 1099

12. Cabot R (1914) *What Men Live By: Work, Play, Love, Worship*. Houghton, Miffin Co, Boston

13. Donaldson LJ (1994) Doctors with problems in an NHS workforce. *Br Med J* **308**: 1277–82

Chapter 15
PRIVATE PRACTICE

◆ Advantages
◆ Disadvantages
◆ Deciding on fees
◆ Other practical considerations

Appointment as an NHS consultant in a clinical specialty carries with it the opportunity of undertaking private practice. I am not going to discuss the contention that private practice is wrong in principle. I fully accept the criticism that it can be abused; and that it has been abused, sometimes seriously. On the other hand, I am impressed by two facts. The first is that it has repeatedly been shown that a substantial majority both of the public and of the profession want private practice to remain. The second is that eminent clinical academics, in both medicine and surgery, who do no private practice themselves, nevertheless support it in principle[1]. Several of them have stated that the standard of service rendered by their colleagues who combine NHS work with private practice is at least as high as that of those who work full time in the Health Service. In addition, they have found that such consultants enrich the quality of both clinical work in hospital and the teaching of medical students.

Advantages

Private practice prevents the NHS from being a monopoly, and provides for patients who want something more than expert diagnosis and treatment. Private patients are often able to see the consultant sooner than they could under the NHS, and to arrange dates for consultation which are more convenient for them, and which minimise loss of earnings.

Several patients came to see me privately because they found the pace of the hospital clinic too hurried, and were disappointed to find that there was no time to ask the doctor the questions they wanted answered. If a patient asked to see me privately because he had not received satisfaction at my hospital clinic, I arranged a fresh NHS outpatient appointment for him and promised to see him there myself.

Personally, I can confirm what many engaged in private practice have said, namely that there is a higher level of job satisfaction in private practice than in the NHS. One of the main reasons for this is that the doctor can give as much time as he wishes to the patient. In a NHS outpatient clinic, a large number of patients have to be seen in a given time, in order to keep down the waiting time for outpatient appointments in the specialty. The duration of the clinic cannot, as a rule, be extended because it would keep nurses, receptionists and other members of staff working late. The current rate of consultation in a typical NHS internal medicine clinic is around five new and 12 follow-up cases within three hours, whereas in private practice I allowed 45 minutes for a new patient and at least 15 minutes for a follow-up patient.

Another advantage of private practice is the satisfaction of knowing that the patient has come to see you rather than anyone else because that was his choice (on the advice of his general practitioner), and that you can see him again personally by mutual agreement. In private practice, one undoubtedly meets some outstandingly interesting patients, including some from overseas, who are ineligible for NHS treatment.

There are also other advantages. The doctor in private practice can get a letter sent to the patient's general practitioner that same day, if necessary. He can also make time to write to the patient personally. Moreover, he can decide the 'tone' and amenities of the waiting room. For example, I had a framed motto from the Bible on display in the waiting room, and included magazines with a spiritual flavour among the usual secular publications. I wanted my patients to realise that I took a holistic view of medical consultation.

Disadvantages

There are potential disadvantages and dangers of private care. It has to be admitted that, in general, inpatient care in a private bed is not as safe as under the NHS. This is because the consultant has to do most of the routine work, and does not have the benefit of the detailed checking of the history and examination ordinarily undertaken by the junior staff. Furthermore, help is less readily available in an emergency. The patient's specialist may be working elsewhere; and if another doctor is available in the hospital, he is unlikely to know the patient as well as the one who had been responsible for clerking him. It is important for doctors to recognise the dangers of making some patients more special than others'[2].

Private practice can be difficult and demanding. Some patients waste the doctor's time. But if so, one can then charge a hefty fee and not see them again.

Practicalities

In private practice, things do not just happen; the consultant has to set them up. He needs premises, including, if possible, four separate rooms, a waiting room, a consulting room, an examination room and a room for his secretary-receptionist.

Doctors are not allowed to advertise their services directly to the public. However, a consultant may circulate his name, qualifications, telephone number, specialty and availability to his consultant colleagues and to local general practitioners. But he must not claim superiority in any way. Initially, some patients will come as family doctors try the new consultant out. After that, the growth of one's practice often depends more on social contacts than on anything else[3].

Deciding on fees

Right at the start, there is a decision to be made regarding the level of fees to be charged. In my view, it is important to charge amounts which are in line with the practice of other consultants in the area. The Monopolies and Mergers Commission investigating private medical services has recently decided that consultants operate a 'complex monopoly'[4]. The BMA guidelines are said to recommend fees 60% higher than those in America and 170% higher than those in France[5]. This issue is not yet resolved.

In the meantime, the advice of Marshall[6] still stands, and I quote it at length with his permission.

> *"The assessment of a reasonable fee is undoubtedly best made on the basis of what is current practice among one's colleagues. If, however, a doctor wishes to charge more than the average, for example to restrict the amount of his private work, he may legitimately do so on two conditions. Firstly, there must be alternative medical services available to those who would consult him, and secondly the patient and any referring practitioner should be aware beforehand of the higher scale of fees. Under these circumstances, patients who do not wish to pay can easily go elsewhere. In the event of the doctor having a monopoly, either because of a special skill, or because there is no other practitioner in the area, he would do wrong to charge more than the fee that is customary in such circumstances; for this would be exploiting his monopoly at the expense of his patients."*

Marshall went on to say:

> *"The doctor must not involve the patient or the Health Service in unnecessary expense. Thus, when it is not strictly necessary either to visit or advise investigation or undertake surgical procedures, it would be wrong to do these things simply because they will be paid for. A*

reasonable interpretation must, of course, be applied when determining what is necessary. The state of a patient's illness may not require a visit, yet the patient may gain great encouragement from the visit of the doctor; it is right to visit for this reason, because it is the whole man and not only his illness that is being treated. Similarly, a doctor may know that a particular investigation is not necessary for diagnosis, but undertakes it because of the reassuring effect it will have on an anxious patient. The illness may not require the investigation, but the patient certainly does. The conscientious doctor knows full well when he is working for the patient's good and when for his own financial gain."

There is also a decision to be made with regard to the waiving of fees for certain categories of patient. A recent survey in America sampled 4800 practising physicians, of whom 2224 responded. Of the respondents, 96% offered 'professional courtesy', defined as free or discounted health care to physicians and their families, although only 80% of psychiatrists did so[7]. I am not aware of any comparable survey of British practice. Personally, I never charged medical or nursing colleagues or their dependants (unless they specifically asked me to submit an account on the grounds that they would be reimbursed); nor did I charge ministers of religion, rendering the service 'pro Deo'. I charged school teachers about half the normal amount. In this matter of fees, the practice of the profession has varied over the years. Formerly, doctors did charge ministers of religion. In one of Somerset Maugham's novels, a vicar complains bitterly about the amount his doctor charged him.

It is important to avoid a reputation for being grasping in money matters, and to be generous to juniors who help in the care of private patients. Scrupulous honesty is vital. It is clearly wrong to use NHS facilities to investigate or treat a private patient or to ask an NHS secretary to type a letter in hospital time. If in doubt about the correct etiquette, it is a wise plan to ask the advice of one of the senior consultants in the region. Such an enquiry will seldom be taken amiss; indeed, most doctors feel flattered to be asked for their advice.

Other practical considerations

One or two more things need to be said. The first is that watertight provision needs to be made for any emergency arising among one's private patients. In the NHS, there is, in principle, round-the-clock medical cover. In private practice, it all depends on the consultant. The general practitioner and the nursing staff need to know where to contact you, and what to do if you are not available. It is important to have an effective partnership or cross-cover with colleagues. Failure at this point can be disastrous.

Consultants in private practice are not covered by NHS insurance for their private work. This must be arranged through one of the defence societies. It is also wise to take out insurance against accidents on the private premises.

The question arises: should a specialist treat a friend as a private patient? Osler is reported to have warned: *"Never make friends with your patients."* A small survey of general practitioners' experiences[8] showed that most of them had friends as patients, and half found the relationship a rewarding one. There were, however, problems. The doctor tended to feel that he was always on call. He also found it difficult to assess situations dispassionately. Other problems included the performance of intimate examinations and the difficulty in maintaining confidentiality, particularly with the patient's spouse.

On retirement from practice, it has been recommended that personal health records should be retained for eight years after the last consultation (Department of Health Circular HC(89)20), to cover the possibility of personal injury claims being brought.

References

1.   Black D (1994) The NHS: a business or service? Threatened values. *Proc. R Coll Physicians Edinb* **24**: 7–14

2.   Dearlove JC (1994) Treatment of doctors' wives (letter). *Br Med J* **309**: 1443

3.   Young AE (1987) Start in private practice. *Br Med J* **295**: 593–4

4.   Smith R (1993) Doctors and Markets. *Br Med J* **307**: 216–7

5.   The Times (London) (1994), 'Consultants' overcharging to be halted' 12 February, p??

6.   Marshall J (1960) *The Ethics of Medical Practice*. Darton, Longman and Todd, London

7.   ABCD (1993) Professional courtesy — current practices and attitudes. *N Engl J Med* **329**: 1627–31

8.   Smith F (1993) Patients as friends (letter). *Br Med J* **306**: 1543

Index